KU-548-370

NURSING85 BOOKS™

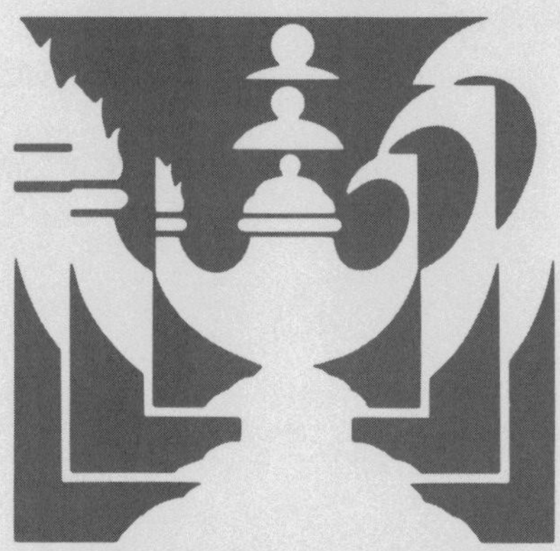

NURSING NOW™ SERIES
Shock
Hypertension
Drug Interactions
Cardiac Crises
Respiratory Emergencies
Pain

NURSING PHOTOBOOK™ SERIES
Providing Respiratory Care
Managing I.V. Therapy
Dealing with Emergencies
Giving Medications
Assessing Your Patients
Using Monitors
Providing Early Mobility
Giving Cardiac Care
Performing GI Procedures
Implementing Urologic Procedures
Controlling Infection
Ensuring Intensive Care
Coping with Neurologic Disorders
Caring for Surgical Patients
Working with Orthopedic Patients
Nursing Pediatric Patients
Helping Geriatric Patients
Attending Ob/Gyn Patients
Aiding Ambulatory Patients
Carrying Out Special Procedures

NEW NURSING SKILLBOOK™ SERIES
Giving Emergency Care Competently
Monitoring Fluid and Electrolytes Precisely
Assessing Vital Functions Accurately
Coping with Neurologic Problems Proficiently
Reading EKGs Correctly
Combatting Cardiovascular Diseases Skillfully
Nursing Critically Ill Patients Confidently
Dealing with Death and Dying
Managing Diabetics Properly
Giving Cardiovascular Drugs Safely

NURSE'S REFERENCE LIBRARY®
Diseases
Diagnostics
Drugs
Assessment
Procedures
Definitions
Practices
Emergencies

***Nursing85* DRUG HANDBOOK™**

NURSE'S CLINICAL LIBRARY™
Cardiovascular Disorders
Respiratory Disorders
Endocrine Disorders
Neurologic Disorders
Renal and Urologic Disorders
Gastrointestinal Disorders
Neoplastic Disorders
Immune Disorders

NURSING NOW™

PAIN

NURSING85 BOOKS™
SPRINGHOUSE CORPORATION
SPRINGHOUSE, PENNSYLVANIA

NURSING NOW™ SERIES

CLINICAL CONSULTANTS FOR THIS VOLUME

Richard Payne, MD
Assistant Attending Neurologist, Memorial Sloan-Kettering Cancer Center, New York

Helen M. Lower, RN, PhD
Director of Undergraduate Nursing, Northwestern University, Chicago

NN6-010185

Library of Congress Cataloging in Publication Data

Main entry under title:
Pain.

(Nursing now)
"Nursing85 books."
Includes bibliographies and index.
1. Pain—Nursing. I. Series: Nursing now series. [DNLM: 1. Pain—nursing. WY 100 P144]
RT87.P35P32 1985 616'.0472 84-26727
ISBN 0-916730-81-6

CONTENTS

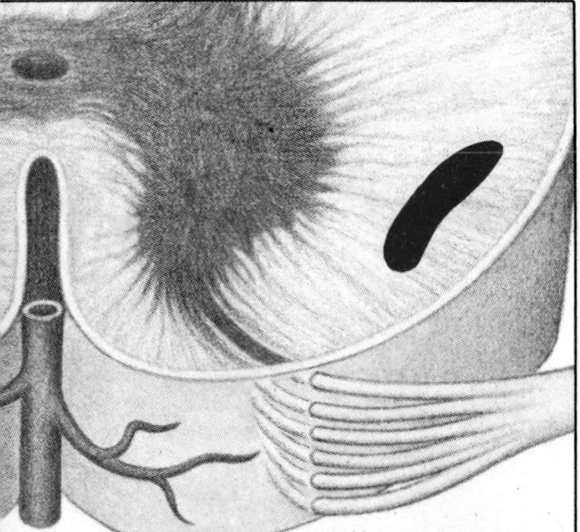

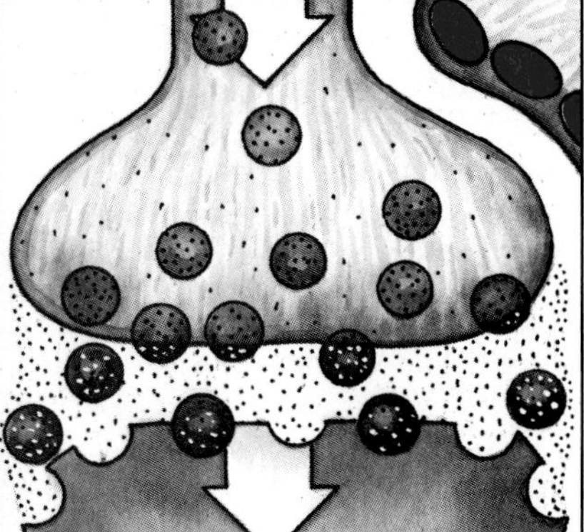

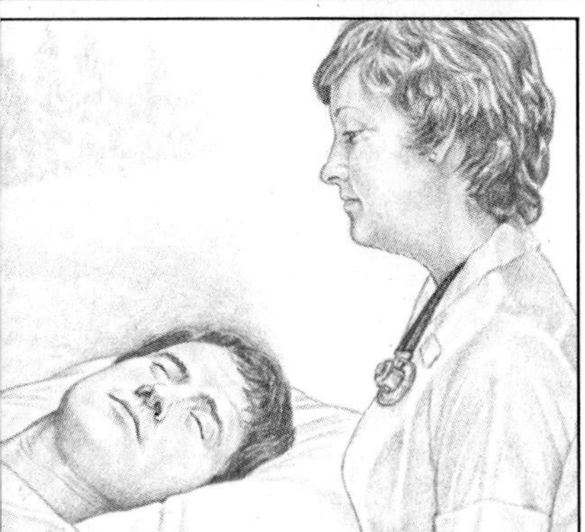

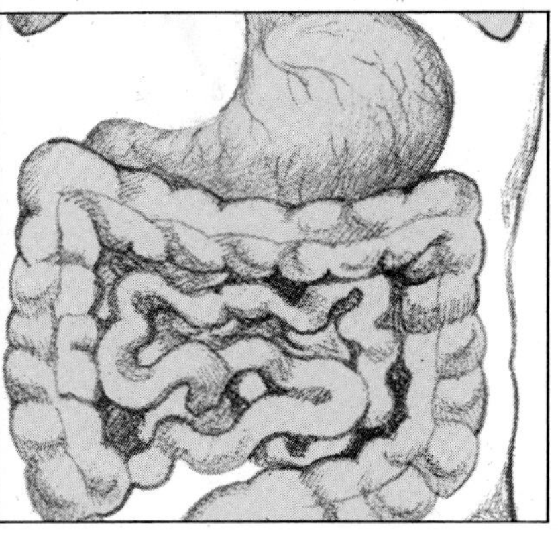

FUNDAMENTALS
MICHELE BOCKRATH, RN, MSN

6 Basic concepts
8 Anatomy
12 Pain transmission
14 Endorphins
16 Pain theories
18 Pain responses
19 Psychosocial factors

ASSESSMENT
CAROLINE STOKES BAGLEY, RN, MSN

26 First steps
30 History
33 Documentation
36 Care plans

NONPHARMACOLOGIC THERAPIES
JENNIFER SUE HOWELL, RN
MARCIA L. LUNA, RN, MN, CS
CHRISTINE A. MIASKOWSKI, RN, MS

38 Basic concepts
41 Conflicts
43 Cognitive strategies
44 Distraction
46 Relaxation
48 Guided imagery
50 Hypnosis
51 Heat and cold
55 Massage
57 T.E.N.S.
60 Biofeedback
62 Acupuncture
64 Alternative therapies
66 Nerve blocks
67 Surgery
70 Pain-control centers

DRUG THERAPY
NESSA COYLE, RN, C, MS
MARGO MCCAFFERY, RN, MS, FAAN

74 Pharmacokinetics
76 Analgesia
78 N.S.A.I.D.s
83 Narcotics
87 Morphine
88 Other narcotics
92 Adjuvant drugs
94 Placebos
97 Analgesic guidelines
102 Special infusion systems

PEDIATRICS
JO ELAND, RN, PhD

108 Primary concerns
111 Assessment
116 Intervention

119 Appendix
125 References and acknowledgments
126 Index

CONTRIBUTORS

At the time of publication, these contributors held the following positions:

Caroline Stokes Bagley is a research nurse specialist in breast cancer at the National Cancer Institute, National Institutes of Health, Bethesda, Maryland. She received her nursing diploma from St. Luke's Hospital in New York, her BSN from Columbia Union College, Takoma Park, Maryland, and her MSN from the Catholic University of America, Washington, D.C. Currently, she's a doctoral candidate at Johns Hopkins University, School of Hygiene and Public Health. Ms. Bagley is a member of the American Nurses' Association, the Council of Nurse Researchers, and the Oncology Nursing Society.

Michele Bockrath is an assistant professor at the University of Delaware in Newark. She received her BSN from the University of Delaware and her MSN from the University of Pennsylvania. She's currently a doctoral student at the University of Maryland. Ms. Bockrath is past president of the Delaware Nurses' Association and is a member of the American Association of Critical-Care Nurses.

Nessa Coyle is director of supportive care, neurology department, pain service, at Memorial Sloan-Kettering Cancer Center, New York. A graduate of St. Bartholomew's Hospital, London, she received her BSN from Cornell University School of Nursing, New York, and her MS as a certified adult nurse practitioner from Columbia University School of Nursing, New York. Ms. Coyle is a member of the Eastern Pain Society, the American Pain Society, and the International Association for the Study of Pain.

Jo Eland is an assistant professor at the University of Iowa, College of Nursing, Iowa City. In addition to her BSN, she earned an MA in the nursing of children and a PhD in educational psychology from the University of Iowa, Iowa City. Ms. Eland is a member of the International Association for the Study of Pain.

Jennifer Sue Howell, an ambulatory administrative nurse, acts as head nurse and clinic manager at the University of Cincinnati Hospital–Pain Control Center, Cincinnati, where she has a joint appointment with the departments of nursing and anesthesiology. She earned her associate nursing degree from the University of Kentucky in Lexington; currently, she's working toward her BSN through New York's regency program. Ms. Howell is a member of the Ohio Nurses Association, the Southwest Ohio Nurses Association, the American Nurses' Association, and the American Pain Society. She's also director-at-large for the Midwest Pain Society.

Helen M. Lower, an advisor for this book, is director of undergraduate nursing at Northwestern University, Chicago. In addition to holding a PhD, she has a BS in nursing and an MS in rehabilitation nursing; she earned them all at State University of New York at Buffalo. Ms. Lower is a member of the American Nurses' Association and the Biofeedback Society of Illinois.

Marcia L. Luna is a mental health clinical nurse specialist at UCLA Medical Center, Los Angeles. She received her BS and MN from the UCLA School of Nursing.

Margo McCaffery is a consultant in the nursing care of patients with pain in Santa Monica, California. She holds a BS from Baylor University, Waco, Texas, and an MS from Vanderbilt University in Nashville. Ms. McCaffery is a Fellow of the American Academy of Nursing (FAAN).

Christine A. Miaskowski is a clinical nurse specialist at the Hospital of the Albert Einstein College of Medicine, New York. She received her BSN from Molloy College, Rockville Center, New York, and her MS from Adelphi University, Garden City, New York. Ms. Miaskowski is a member of the American Pain Society, the International Association for the Study of Pain, and the Oncology Nursing Society.

Richard Payne, an advisor for this book, is an assistant attending neurologist at Memorial Sloan-Kettering Cancer Center, New York. A graduate of Harvard Medical School, Dr. Payne is a member of the American Academy of Neurology, the American Pain Society, and the International Association for the Study of Pain.

FUNDAMENTALS

BASIC CONCEPTS
ANATOMY
PAIN TRANSMISSION
ENDORPHINS
PAIN THEORIES
PAIN RESPONSES
PSYCHOSOCIAL FACTORS

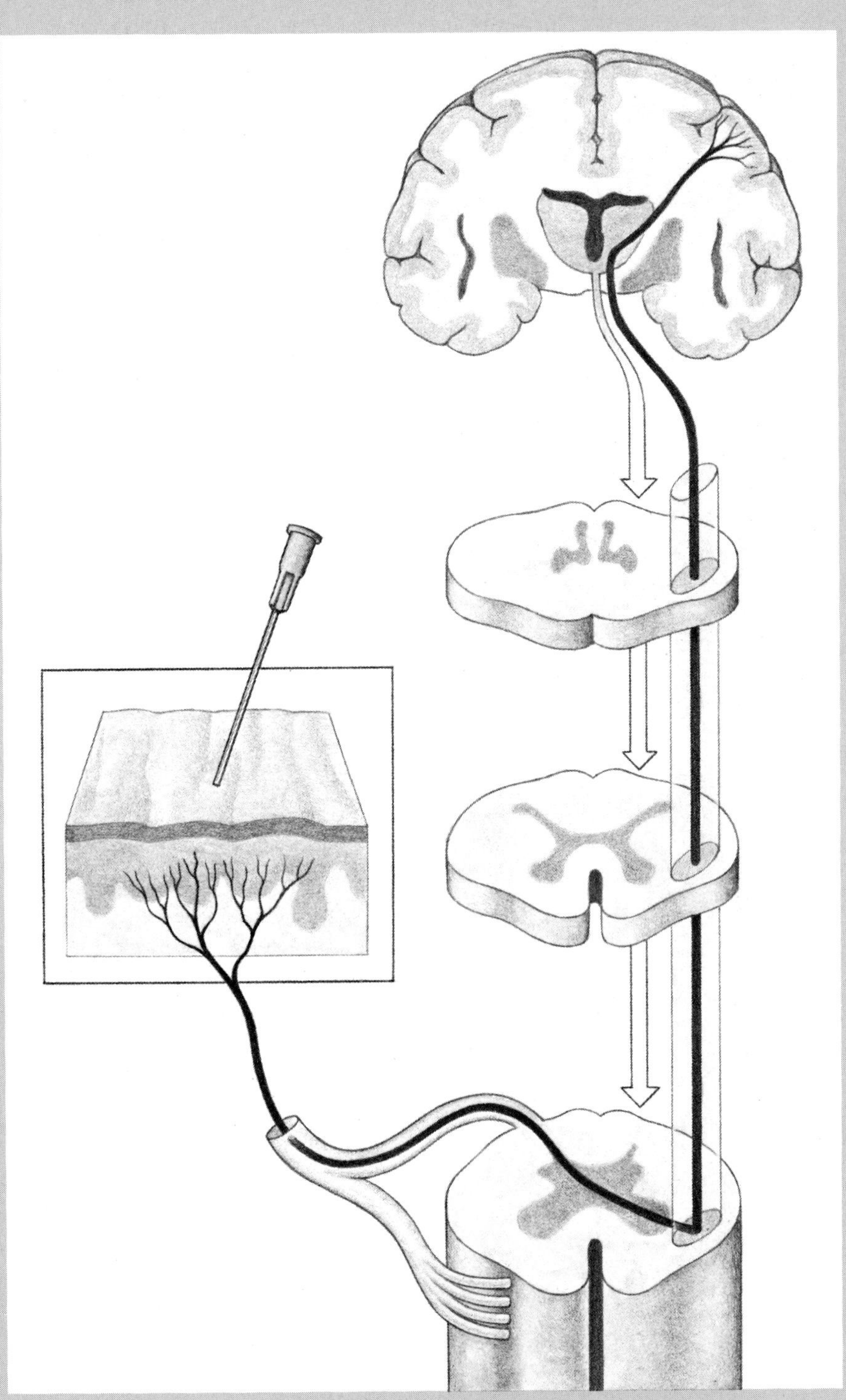

BASIC CONCEPTS

PAIN: A FACT OF LIFE

Pain is one of life's paradoxes: On one hand, it's a universal phenomenon that everyone experiences at least occasionally during life. Yet it's so personal and private that each person's experience is unique. The sufferer himself is the only true expert on his pain.

In its many forms, ranging from sharp stabs to dull aches, pain demands attention—sometimes to the exclusion of all other considerations. The word itself derives from the Greek word for *penalty*, suggesting an ancient perception of pain as a price we pay for living.

Of course, pain isn't designed as random punishment. Rather, it's a primal warning system that protects against injury and encourages immobilization during healing. Although acute pain can be excruciating, it's usually both transient and purposeful. But when pain becomes chronic, it loses meaning and threatens well-being.

Despite pain's universality, it's an incompletely understood phenomenon that's usually discussed in terms of theory, not fact. Physiology and perception are so tightly intertwined that distinguishing one element from the other is sometimes impossible. One result of our confusion is that pain—whether acute or chronic—is often inadequately managed, to the detriment of our patients who suffer.

In this book, we'll sort out current thinking on what pain is, how it occurs, and what factors influence pain perception. In addition, we'll explore proven and promising pain-control strategies. By learning more about pain, you'll be better equipped to help relieve suffering—the oldest and most important of your nursing responsibilities.

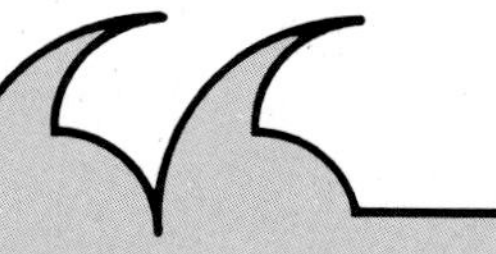

"All pain is real, regardless of its cause. Pain is whatever the person experiencing it says it is and exists whenever he says it does.

"Unfortunately, some health-care professionals erroneously believe that if emotions cause or perpetuate pain, the pain is imaginary and thus not real. But calling pain imaginary won't make it go away. No pain sensation is truly imaginary—certainly not to the patient. You must believe that his pain is real before you can help him."

Margo McCaffery, RN, MS, FAAN
Consultant in the Nursing Care of Patients with Pain
Santa Monica, Calif.

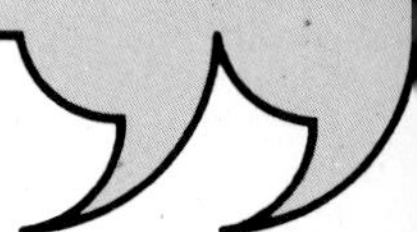

ACUTE VERSUS CHRONIC PAIN: HOW THEY DIFFER

Although you may be inclined to think of chronic pain as an extension of acute pain, the two pain types differ significantly in many ways. Throughout this book, you'll see how assessment and intervention are influenced by the type of pain involved.

By definition, acute pain lasts less than 6 months; chronic pain, more than 6 months. But because the point at which acute pain becomes chronic varies among patients, the considerations in this chart may provide a better guide than this arbitrary time frame.

	ACUTE	CHRONIC
Location	May be highly localized	May be poorly localized
Characteristics	Usually sharp; may radiate. Generally arises from an acute injury or disease process and passes quickly	Dull, aching, diffuse, constant, nagging; may be intractable. May be associated with chronic pathology, or may persist after recovery from a disease or injury
Signs and symptoms	Associated with autonomic nervous system (ANS) response: increased blood pressure, tachycardia, diaphoresis, pallor, mydriasis, restlessness, grimacing facial expression, anxiety	ANS signs and symptoms may be absent; patient may appear exhausted, listless, depressed, and withdrawn
Patient expectations	Patient may expect intervention to relieve pain	Patient may expect intervention to reduce pain but also expects pain to continue

PAIN COMPONENTS

What constitutes pain? Because it's an individually perceived process, each pain experience is shaped by the sufferer's unique physiology, emotions, and life experiences. In this section, we'll explore pain's many facets in detail. In the meantime, keep these considerations in mind.

• *Physiology.* Although each individual has the same basic physiologic makeup, distinct physical differences make some people more (or less) susceptible to pain than others. Some people have a rare congenital defect that makes them totally insensitive to pain.

• *Personal and cultural attitudes.* In some cultures, pain is considered a punishment to be endured stoically. In others, pain is openly expressed and even dramatized. Similarly, individuals are affected by their values and priorities. A professional football player, for example, may consider pain to be a fact of life that he must accept and try to ignore.

• *Cognitive significance.* What does the pain mean to the individual? In one classic study, wounded soldiers needed far fewer analgesics than did surgical patients with comparable wounds. The reason? The soldiers apparently associated their injuries—and the accompanying pain—with survival and escape from further danger.

On the other hand, a patient with terminal cancer may interpret his pain as a reminder of impending death. Similarly, severe, chronic pain (for example, from rheumatoid arthritis) may become inextricably linked to hopelessness and despair.

The five most frequently mentioned pain sites

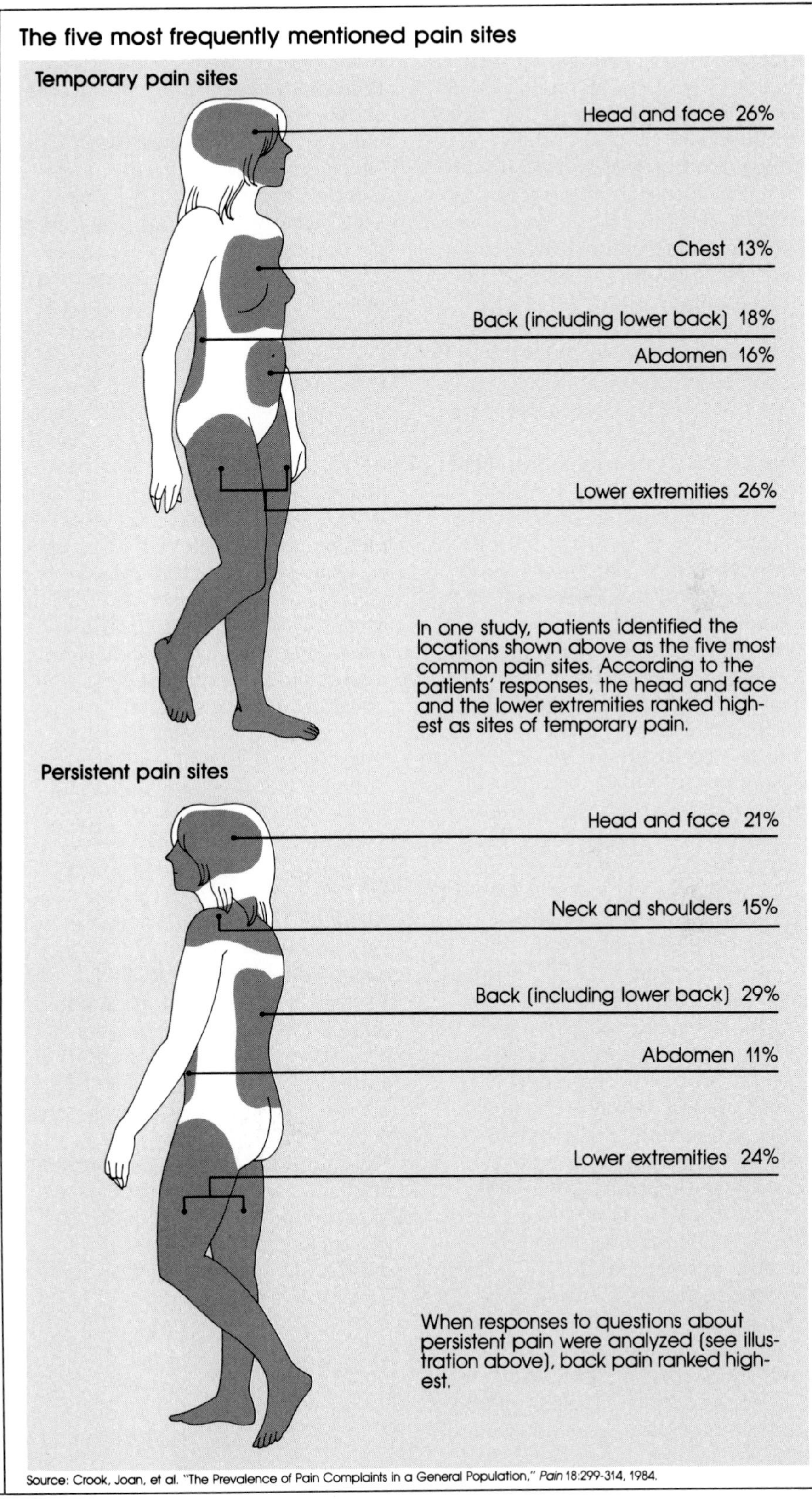

Source: Crook, Joan, et al. "The Prevalence of Pain Complaints in a General Population," *Pain* 18:299-314, 1984.

BASIC CONCEPTS CONTINUED

A GLOSSARY OF TERMS

Before reading further, familiarize yourself with the following common neurologic terms. You'll see them again.

Afferent. Ingoing; traveling toward a center. Sensory neurons, which carry messages to the central nervous system (CNS), are afferent. Dendrites, which gather information for individual neurons, accept afferent impulses from axons.

Axon. A neuron's efferent segment; it conducts impulses away from the cell body.

Dendrites. A neuron's fine, free-branching afferent segments; they conduct impulses to the cell body.

Dermatome. A skin area innervated by sensory neurons that share the same spinal nerve root; each dermatome corresponds to a specific spinal cord level.

Dorsal horn. The posterior portion of the spinal cord's gray matter, to which sensory nerve fibers are attached. Also called the *posterior horn,* the dorsal horn receives sensory impulses from the body and relays them toward the brain.

Efferent. Outgoing; traveling away from a center. Motor neurons, which carry messages away from the CNS, are efferent. An axon, which carries impulses away from the cell body, is a neuron's efferent segment.

Gray matter. Grayish concentration of neuron cell bodies (somata) in the brain and spinal cord. Gray matter also includes proximal portions of axons, neuroglial cells, and capillaries.

Limbic system. An umbrella term for subcortical structures common to all mammals that are involved in autonomic functions, behavior, emotion, and olfaction. Limbic structures, which include the hippocampus, thalamus, and hypothalamus, are believed to play a role in pain modulation.

Myelin. A white, fatty sheath that surrounds some axons and enhances impulse transmission.

Neospinothalamic tract. An ascending spinal cord pathway located in the white matter's lateral portion and leading to the thalamus. This tract is associated with transmission of sharp, well-localized pain and crude touch and pressure sensations.

Neuron. A nerve cell consisting of dendrites, cell body, and axon.

Nociceptors. Pain receptors; free nerve endings sensitive to painful mechanical, thermal, electrical, or chemical stimuli.

Paleospinothalamic tract. An ascending spinal cord pathway leading to the reticular formation of the brain stem and frontal lobe. This tract is associated with transmission of dull, aching, and burning pain sensations.

Substantia gelatinosa. Small, densely packed cells within the dorsal horn involved in pain impulse modulation.

Synapse. The space between neurons (or between a neuron and a muscle or organ) that a nerve impulse must cross for transmission to occur. It's also called the *synaptic cleft.*

Ventral horn. The anterior portion of the spinal cord's gray matter, to which motor (and some sensory) nerve fibers are attached. It's also called the *anterior horn.*

White matter. Tissue surrounding gray matter; composed of axons (primarily), neuroglial cells, and some capillaries. The axons' myelin sheaths give white matter its characteristic color.

ANATOMY

THE NEURON: FIRST STOP ON THE PAIN PATHWAY

The peripheral nervous system (PNS)—which includes spinal motor and sensory nerves and dorsal root ganglion cells—provides a communications network for the CNS. Working together, the PNS and the CNS receive, transmit, and interpret sensory messages—including pain messages—and regulate the body's responses to them.

Two major cell types make up

Motor neuron

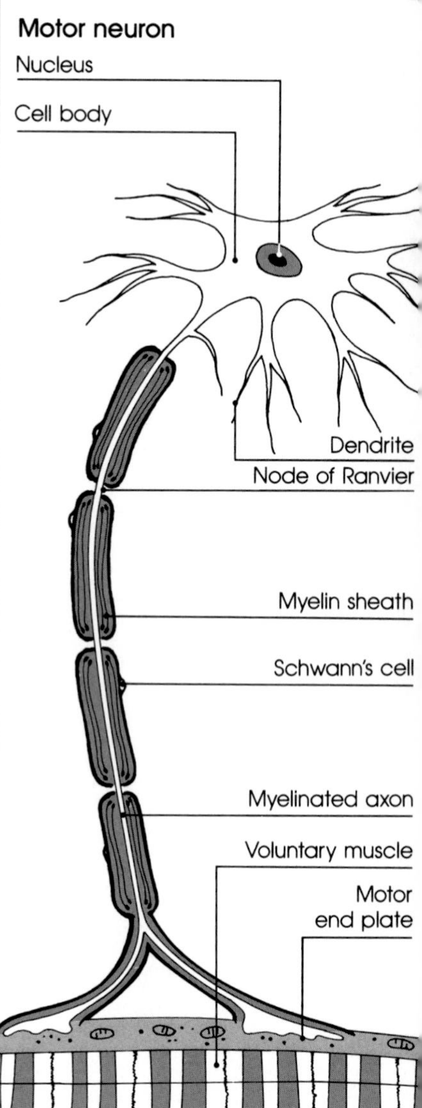

the nervous system: neurons and neuroglial cells. Neuroglial cells are nonexcitable and therefore can't receive or transmit pain messages (for more about them, see page 10). But neurons are on the front line of pain reception and transmission. Let's take a closer look.

Types and characteristics. Neurons can be classified as follows: afferent (sensory) neurons, whose axons transmit impulses to the CNS; efferent (motor) neurons, whose axons transmit impulses from the CNS to other tissues; and interneurons (go-between cells that aid communication between motor and sensory neurons). But despite their functional differences, most neurons share these basic anatomic features:

- a cell body (soma), which contains the cell nucleus
- multiple, branching dendrites, which receive messages from the neuron's environment and communicate them to the cell body
- an axon, which carries impulses away from the cell body. Unlike dendrites, which are relatively short, axons can be quite long—24" (61 cm) or more.

Some axons have a myelin sheath, a lipid coating with regular breaks resembling constrictions called *nodes of Ranvier.* Nerve impulses skip rapidly from node to node by a process called *saltatory conduction.* Because of this conduction process, myelinated axons transmit impulses more quickly than unmyelinated ones.

Fiber types. Based on conduction speed, axons are broadly categorized as A, B, and C fibers. A fibers, which are myelinated, conduct impulses quickest; unmyelinated C fibers, slowest. A fibers are further subgrouped into alpha, beta, gamma, and delta fibers.

Of all these fiber types, only A-delta and C fibers seem involved in pain transmission. A-delta fibers transmit sharp pain sensations. C fibers, which are smaller in diameter, transmit the dull, aching, or burning sensations that follow sharply painful sensations. Pain transmitted by C fibers is less localized but more persistent than pain transmitted by A-delta fibers.

Serotonin, norepinephrine, and substance P appear to be important neurotransmitters involved in pain modulation.

Making a connection. Interaction between two neurons occurs from either electrical or chemical impulse transmission across a synapse. Although the exact mechanism is unclear, chemical transmission may occur when an impulse stimulates release of a neurotransmitter chemical (such as acetylcholine) from vesicles at the neuron terminal. The chemical crosses the synapse to the neighboring neuron, which then responds to the chemical message. The message may stimulate the neuron to carry the impulse further; or it may inhibit the neuron and delay or stop the impulse.

A sampling of neurons

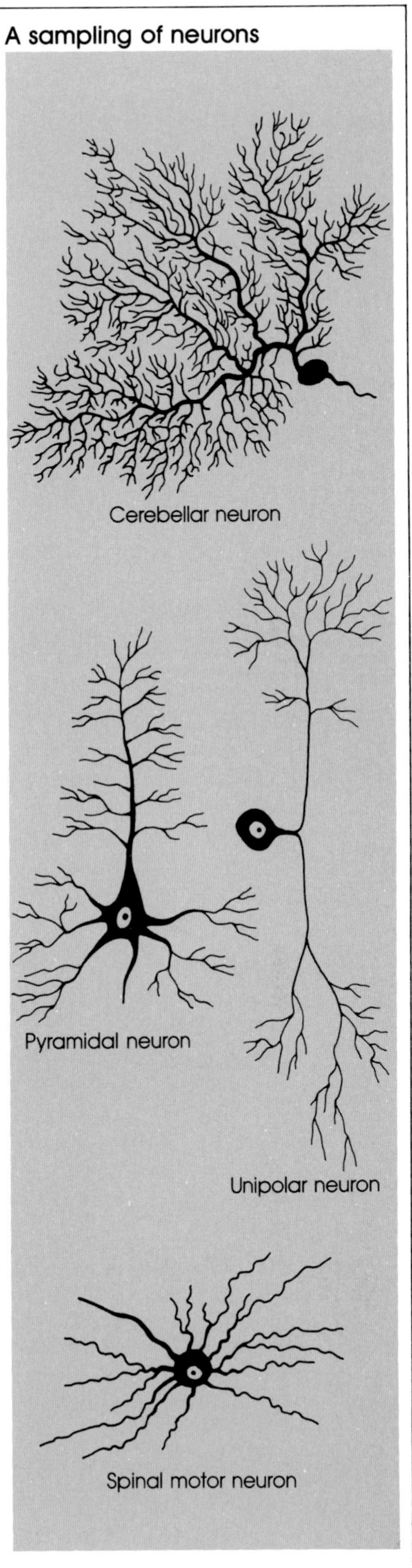

ANATOMY CONTINUED

SENSORY RECEPTOR TYPES

The tips of a sensory neuron's axon serve as sensory receptors that respond to such stimuli as pressure, temperature, electrical energy, and chemical changes. These highly specialized nerve endings respond to one or a few specific stimuli within a narrow range. However, stimulation of one tissue region may activate more than one receptor type. *Note:* Some tissue (for example, the brain and the lungs' alveoli) apparently have no pain receptors at all.

In general, receptors are classified by location and by the stimulus most likely to activate (or inhibit) them. For example, muscle and tendon receptors involved with joint positioning are called proprioceptors; light-sensitive receptors in the eye's rods and cones are called photoreceptors. And receptors that respond to injury or noxious stimuli are called *nociceptors,* or pain receptors.

How these free, structurally undifferentiated nerve endings sense pain is unclear. One likely explanation is that substances released in response to injury—for example, bradykinin, histamine, proteolytic enzymes, and prostaglandins—increase pain sensitivity by lowering the stimulation threshold of nociceptors. When stimulated, nociceptors generate an afferent impulse, which causes release of neurotransmitter chemicals (such as the peptide substance P). These chemicals, in turn, transmit (or inhibit) impulse transmission.

Unlike other sensory receptors, nociceptors don't become less sensitive if stimulation persists. Instead, they may become *more* sensitive, resulting in continuous pain after such serious injuries as burns or other trauma.

Although all nociceptors are structurally similar, they respond differently to noxious stimuli, according to their location in the body. For example, a cutting injury causes acute pain in the skin but not in the viscera. Similarly, moderate stretching causes pain in the viscera but not in the skin.

NEUROGLIAL CELLS

Although not directly involved in the transmission of pain and other sensations, the three types of neuroglial cells provide important support for the CNS. More numerous than neurons, neuroglial cells aid communication between neurons and perform other integrative functions. Depending on specific cell type, these functions include:

- making and maintaining myelin; conveying nutrients and wastes between neurons and blood vessels or cerebrospinal fluid (CSF)
- making repairs after trauma; acting as phagocytes at injury sites
- lining the upper portions of the CNS, confining CSF.

Unlike neurons, neuroglial cells may reproduce rapidly after CNS injury. Some CNS tumors result from pathologic overgrowth of neuroglial cells.

FROM SPINAL CORD TO BRAIN

In itself, stimulation of nociceptors doesn't cause pain. Pain results only when the pain message is relayed to the brain, which then interprets the message. The spinal cord is the bridge between the pain impulse and the brain.

For a close look at the spinal cord, examine the cross section illustrated on the following page. As you see, the cord has an internal, butterfly-shaped mass of gray matter surrounded by white matter. The gray matter is divided into areas called horns. Sensory (afferent) nerve fibers enter the posterior, or dorsal, horns: motor (efferent) fibers exit from the anterior, or ventral, horns. The dorsal and ventral horns thus anchor the roots of each spinal nerve.

Once they reach the dorsal horns, sensory impulses travel to the brain along specialized tracts. Pain impulses travel up the lateral spinothalamic tract to the thalamus, which disseminates the message to other parts of the brain.

Although researchers once believed that pain impulses stimulated a specific pain center in the brain, they now know that virtually all parts of the brain can influence pain perception.

The limbic system, which includes the hypothalamus and parts of the frontal lobe, may play an important role in pain perception, especially pain's emotional, suffering component.

Cross section of the spinal cord

When viewed cross-sectionally, the spinal cord consists of gray matter—including the ventral (anterior) and dorsal (posterior) horns—surrounded by white matter. As shown below, a segment of each dorsal horn is called the *substantia gelatinosa;* this tissue is especially important to pain-impulse modulation.

White matter contains many nerve fiber tracts that relay messages to and from the brain. In this illustration, we've identified the *lateral spinothalamic tracts,* which are ascending pain pathways. Learn more about them on the next two pages.

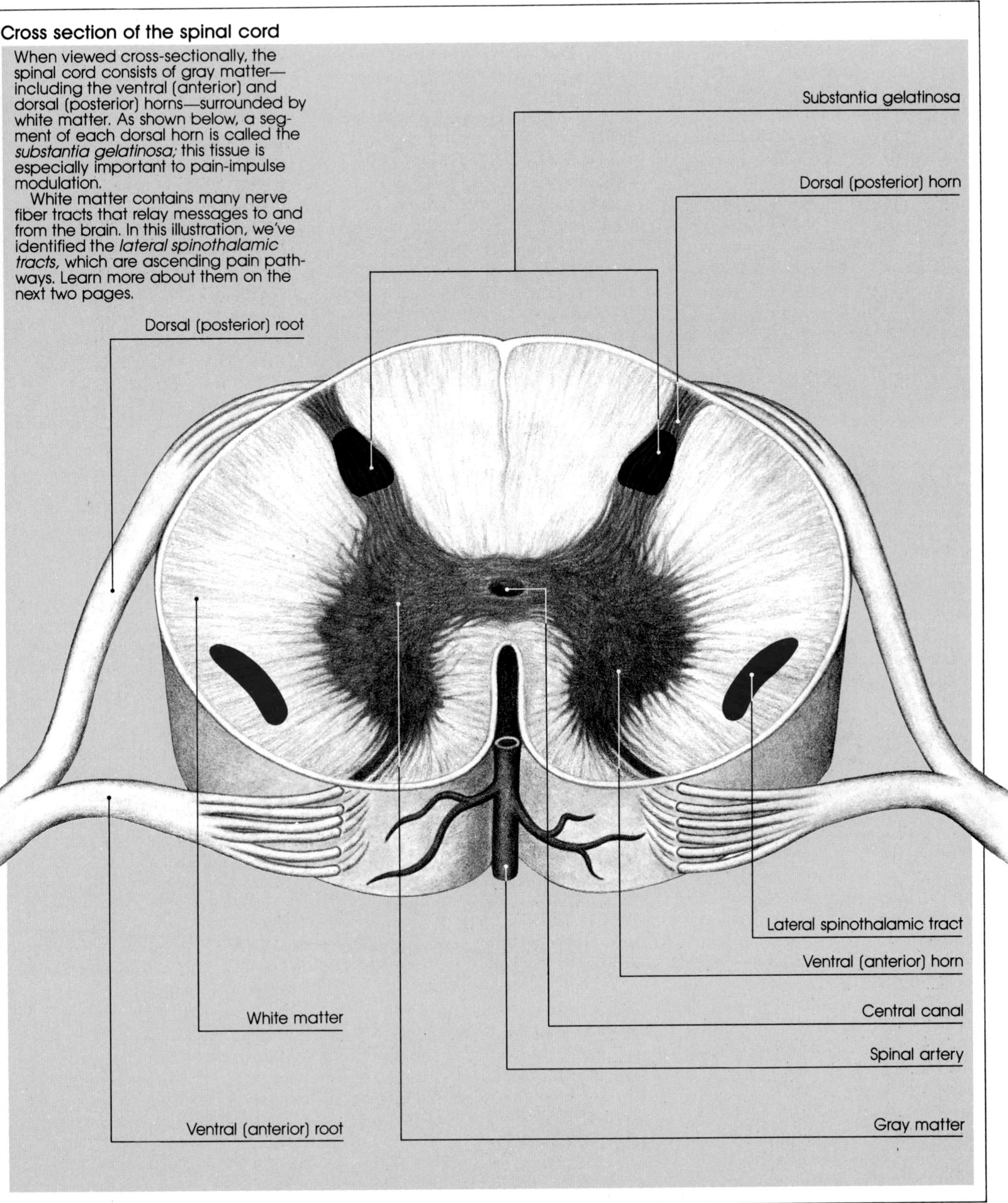

PAIN TRANSMISSION

PAIN REGULATORS

Pain impulses are regulated in part by endogenous substances that act at various points along the pain pathways. These regulators can be classified as follows:

Algogenic substances. After an injury, the body releases or produces pain-producing (algogenic) substances that increase the irritability of pain receptors and initiate pain impulses. These locally released substances include histamine, bradykinin (and other kinins), serotonin, and prostaglandins.

During the inflammatory process, serotonin and histamine are directly released from tissues; bradykinin is released from globulin in interstitial fluids; and prostaglandin is synthesized locally at the injury site. Prostaglandins in the tissues sensitize pain receptors and enhance the effects of histamine and bradykinin. Nonsteroidal analgesics such as aspirin relieve pain by inhibiting prostaglandin synthesis.

Neurotransmitters. These substances, which act at the central level, aid or inhibit impulse transmission across synapses. Among the substances proven to be neurotransmitters are acetylcholine, norepinephrine, epinephrine, and dopamine. Other substances, including gamma-aminobutyric acid (GABA), somatostatin, and the peptide substance P (pain), are putative (probable) neurotransmitters. (Some researchers also consider histamine and serotonin to be putative neurotransmitters.)

Substance P may act at the dorsal horn to enhance pain impulse transmission; however, whether or not substance P is specific to pain transmission is controversial. GABA and somatostatin may act to inhibit (not enhance) pain impulse transmission, although this is also controversial. *Note:* Serotonin, which enhances pain transmission at the local level, apparently inhibits pain when it acts on central nervous system structures, such as the dorsal horn and the raphe nuclei of the medulla.

MORE ON PROSTAGLANDINS

Causing pain is only one of the many effects prostaglandins exert throughout the body. These potent fatty acids can stimulate a wide range of sometimes-contradictory effects, including vasodilation, vasoconstriction, and smooth-muscle relaxation or contraction. They also affect renal sodium excretion, electrolyte balance, gastric acid secretion, and body temperature. The specific effect depends on the prostaglandin type and where it's released.

Prostaglandins are synthesized within cells after cell membrane injury. Rather than storing prostaglandins, the cells immediately release them into the environment, where they exert a local effect. They can appear in small quantities almost anywhere in the body. Active for a relatively short time, their half-life is from seconds to minutes.

The type of prostaglandin synthesized depends on the cell that produces it. Prostaglandin types are identified by letter additions to PG (prostaglandin) and a subscript number; PGE_1 and PGE_2, for example, are powerful vasodilators involved in the pain response. Other prostaglandin types are identified by the letters A, B, F, and I. At present, more than 15 prostaglandin types have been identified.

FOLLOWING PAIN PATHWAYS

How do pain impulses get from the peripheral nervous system to the brain? And how does the CNS process the information and respond? Presently, no one has all the answers. However, the following sequence of events is currently the most widely accepted explanation.

From spine to brain. Upon entering the spinal cord through a spinal nerve's dorsal (posterior) root, pain impulses activate neurons in the dorsal horn, which is composed of numerous cell layers (laminae) that extend along each side of the spinal cord. Two of these layers, called the *substantia gelatinosa,* are particularly important in pain transmission and modulation.

Following axons of dorsal horn neurons, the impulses cross to the opposite side of the spinal cord. Then they ascend to the thalamus. From the thalamus, relay fibers carry the impulses to the cerebral cortex and other brain structures.

Several ascending pathways contribute to pain transmission. But the pathway most prominently involved in pain transmission is the lateral spinothalamic tract, which has two parallel subdivisions.

• The *neospinothalamic tract,* which ascends in the lateral area of the spinal cord's white matter, leads to the ventrolateral and posterior portions of the thalamus. This tract carries impulses initially transmitted by A-delta peripheral fibers. Because it transmits impulses quickly, it's associated with sharp, well-localized pain. It permits perception of pain location and intensity and triggers such behavioral mechanisms as the fight-or-flight response.

• The *paleospinothalamic tract,*

which transmits impulses initially transmitted by C peripheral fibers, leads to the reticular formation and the thalamus. Impulses traveling this pathway are relayed to the limbic system, among other brain structures. This tract transmits impulses more slowly than the neospinothalamic tract; as a result, it's associated with burning, aching, dull, and poorly localized sensations. Because it affects brain structures that control memory and recall, it's probably involved in emotional responses to pain.

Note: Neither of these tracts carries pain impulses exclusively; for example, the neospinothalamic tract also conveys crude touch and pressure sensations.

Descending pathways. In the brain itself, specific areas control or influence pain perception. The hypothalamus, for example, serves as the emotional center for pain perception; the frontal cortex controls rational interpretation and response to pain. Under some circumstances, the cortex can actually suppress pain.

The brain relays its responses along the lateral and ventral pyramidal and extrapyramidal tracts—descending pathways of efferent fibers that extend from the cerebral cortex and the brain stem down the spinal cord. These descending pathways can inhibit or modify incoming pain impulses by a feedback loop mechanism involving the substantia gelatinosa and other dorsal horn layers. Consequently, descending pathways can influence pain impulses at the spinal level. The gate control theory provides an explanation for this process; we'll examine it in detail on pages 16 to 17.

Ascending and descending pathways

After a stimulus (such as a needle) generates a pain impulse in the skin, neurons carry the impulse to the spinal cord's dorsal (posterior) horn. (In this case, the impulse enters at the cervical spinal level.) The impulse travels to the brain via the lateral spinothalamic tract, which is represented here by a vertical black line. Brain responses travel down the spinal cord along descending pathways, indicated by white arrows.

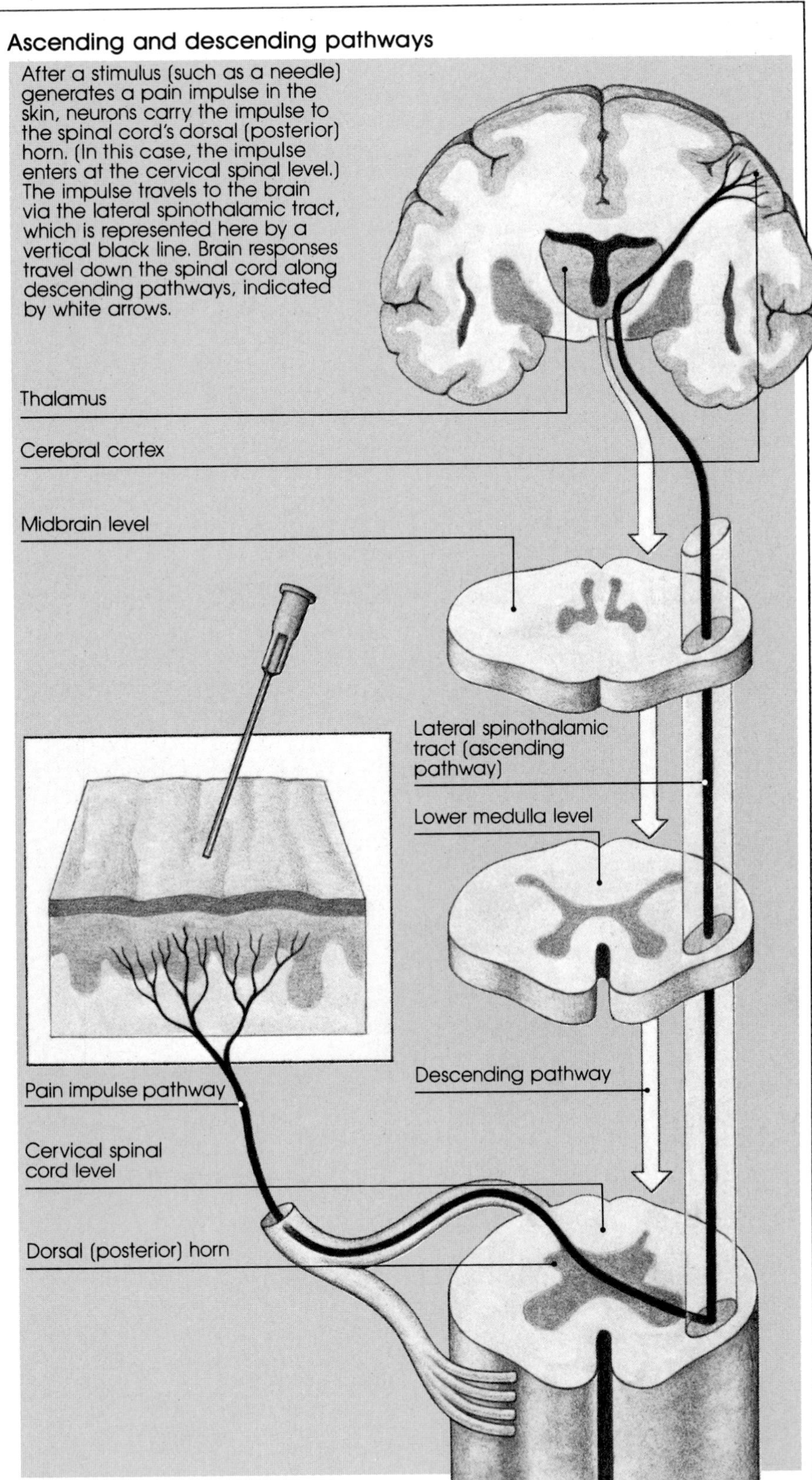

ENDORPHINS

ENDORPHINS AND OTHER ENDOGENOUS OPIOIDS

Endogenous opioid peptides, such as endorphin, are chemical regulators that probably modulate pain through several different mechanisms. By binding with opiate receptor sites throughout the nervous system—particularly in the dorsal horn—they may inhibit release of such neurotransmitters as substance P. In addition, they may alter pain perception.

Currently, endogenous opioids are classified into three major groups:

- *enkephalin* (meaning *in the head*). A small polypeptide, enkephalin binds with opiate receptors in the dorsal horn of the spinal cord, apparently inhibiting the release of substance P; as a result, its effects are weakly analgesic. Outside the spinal cord, it's also concentrated in the brain stem, limbic system, hypothalamus, adrenal glands, and GI tract. (The presence of opiate receptors in the GI tract helps explain why morphine and other narcotics can cause constipation.) *Met-enkephalin* and *leuenkephalin* are subgroups.
- *endorphin* (a combination of the words *endogenous* and *morphine*). A larger polypeptide, endorphin may be synthesized and stored by the pituitary gland; it's also found in the hypothalamus, midbrain, and limbic system. Several subgroups have been identified, including *beta-endorphin*, which is highly concentrated in the hypothalamus and the pituitary gland. Beta-endorphin is a much more potent analgesic than enkephalin.

> *In addition to pain, other types of stress (for example, strenuous, prolonged exercise) can stimulate release of endogenous opioids.*

- *dynorphin* (a combination of the words *dynamite* and *endorphin)*. A more recently discovered compound, dynorphin is found in the pituitary gland, hypothalamus, and spinal cord. Its analgesic effects are 50 times more powerful than those of beta-endorphin.

Such pain-relief therapies as acupuncture, placebos, and transcutaneous electrical nerve stimulation (TENS) may work because they stimulate release of endogenous opioids. One convincing piece of evidence for a connection between acupuncture and endogenous opioid release is that the narcotic antagonist naloxone hydrochloride (Narcan) reverses acupuncture's analgesic effect.

Ideally, analgesic drug therapy would mimic the effects of endogenous opioids without producing unwanted narcotic effects (such as respiratory depression and blood pressure changes). Selective spinal analgesia—epidural injection of morphine, beta-endorphin, or an enkephalin—can produce long-lasting analgesia with few adverse effects. Along the same lines, researchers recently have focused on injecting endorphins directly into the dorsal horn.

How endorphins stop pain transmission

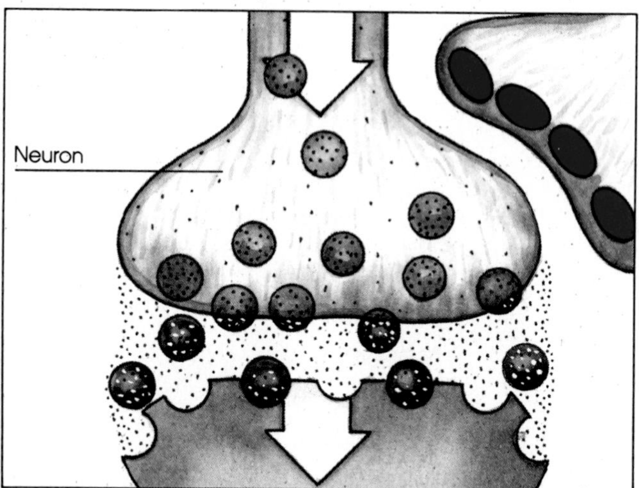

To permit pain-impulse transmission, excitatory sensory neurons release neurotransmitters, illustrated above by gray spheres. By binding to receptors on an adjacent neuron, neurotransmitters perpetuate the pain impulse.

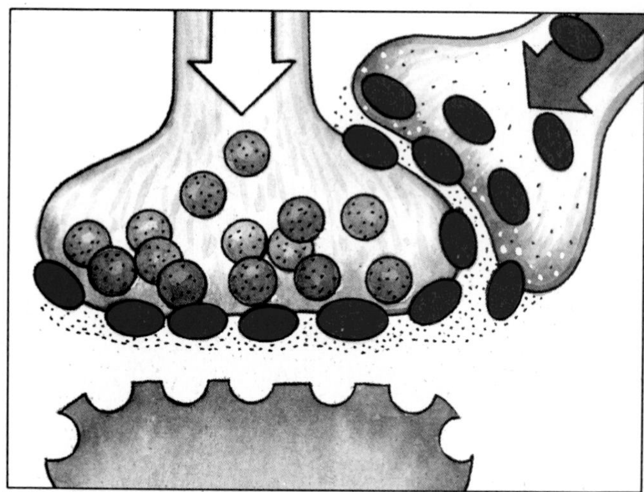
In this illustration, an inhibitory neuron has released endorphins, represented by colored ovals. By binding to receptor sites on the excitatory neuron, endorphins prevent neurotransmitter release and halt the pain impulse.

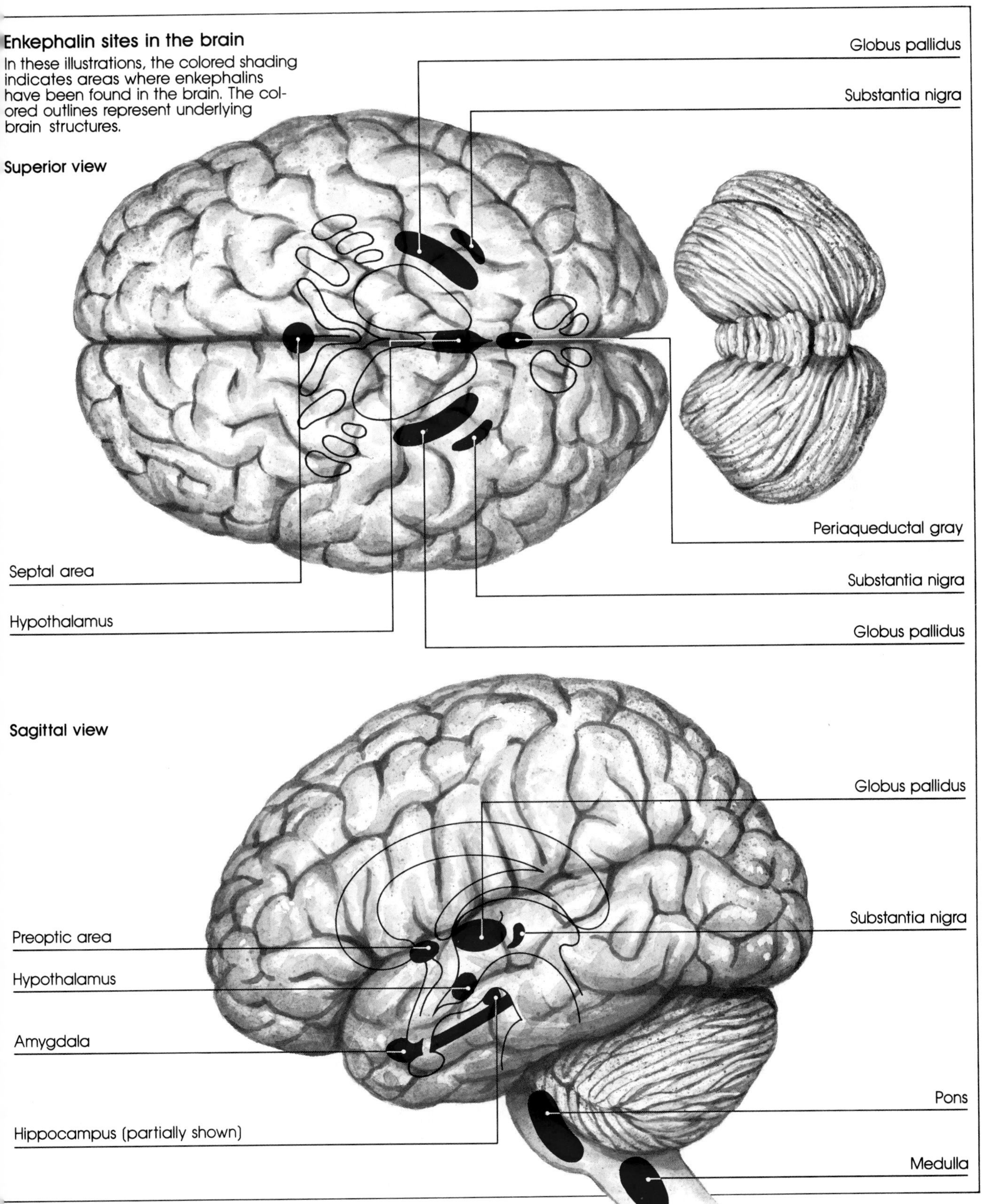
Enkephalin sites in the brain
In these illustrations, the colored shading indicates areas where enkephalins have been found in the brain. The colored outlines represent underlying brain structures.
Superior view
Globus pallidus
Substantia nigra
Periaqueductal gray
Septal area
Substantia nigra
Hypothalamus
Globus pallidus
Sagittal view
Globus pallidus
Substantia nigra
Preoptic area
Hypothalamus
Amygdala
Pons
Hippocampus (partially shown)
Medulla

PAIN THEORIES

EXPLAINING PAIN

As researchers have learned more about pain physiology, theories designed to explain how and why we feel pain have changed. The *specificity theory,* which dates back at least 200 years, assumes that pain travels from specific pain receptors to a pain center in the brain and that the relationship between a pain stimulus and pain response is direct, uniform, and invariable. Although a useful explanation for how pain travels along pain pathways, the specificity theory has some flaws:

- It assumes that specific fibers carry only pain impulses; we now know that pain, pressure, and temperature sensations travel along the same fibers.
- It assumes a direct relationship between stimulus intensity and perceived pain, even though the same stimulus may evoke different responses in different people—or even in the same person, under different circumstances.
- It assumes that only one brain structure responds to the pain impulses; we now know that many parts of the brain are involved and that a specific pain center probably doesn't exist.
- It doesn't explain how sensation can progress from a pleasant to a painful feeling; for example, from pleasantly warm to painfully hot.
- It doesn't account for the psychological component of pain.

Another theory. To deal with some of the specificity theory's limitations, researchers developed the *pattern theory*—actually a combination of several similar concepts. According to the pattern theory, pain impulses generated by receptors form a pattern, or code, that informs the CNS that pain is present.

One of this theory's key concepts is that nerve fiber circuits can become established in groups of spinal interneurons following an injury, causing ongoing pain even without stimulation. Called a *reverberating circuit,* this mechanism could explain such phenomena as phantom limb pain. But such procedures as cordotomy—which would presumably sever a reverberating circuit—usually don't relieve pain permanently, suggesting that other mechanisms are also involved.

Gate control. First proposed in 1965, the gate control theory borrows elements from the specificity theory and the pattern theory. Although controversial and subject to ongoing revision, gate control is currently one of the most widely accepted pain theories. We'll examine it in more detail at right.

"No single theory—be it specificity, pattern, or gate control—comprehensively explains the way the nervous system processes nociceptive information. As we learn more about pain and pain transmission, we'll probably discover that all three theories have elements that help explain pain perception and modulation."

Richard Payne, MD
Assistant Attending Neurologist
Memorial Sloan-Kettering
Cancer Center
New York

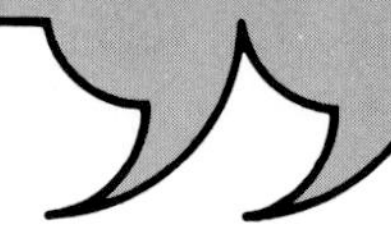

GATE CONTROL: ANOTHER PAIN CONCEPT

Why do such measures as massage and Lamaze breathing provide pain relief for many patients? Why do responses to a painful injury vary widely among individuals? How does acupuncture work? Because the specificity and pattern theories don't adequately answer these and other questions, researchers Ronald Melzack and Patrick Wall developed a more comprehensive view of pain transmission and perception known as the *gate control theory.* Although many of its original assumptions have been disproven, this theory provides the most comprehensive and practical model for conceptualizing pain.

Basic concepts. The premise of gate control is that pain is modulated by a gating mechanism located in the spinal cord as well as by activity in higher CNS structures. Basic assumptions include the following points:

- Afferent (sensory) impulses can travel to the dorsal horn along the large-diameter (A fiber, excluding A-delta fiber) nerves and the small-diameter (A-delta or C fiber) nerves associated with pain impulses.
- At the dorsal horn, the impulses encounter a gate thought to be substantia gelatinosa cells. This gate, which may be presynaptic or postsynaptic, can be open, partially open, or closed. If the gate is closed, pain impulses can't proceed. If the gate is open (or partially open), pain impulses stimulate T (transmission or trigger) cells in the dorsal horn. The impulses then ascend the spinal cord to the brain, and pain perception results (unless a CNS feedback mechanism halts impulse transmission).
- Gate position depends on whether large- or small-fiber im-

pulses predominate. When large-fiber impulses predominate, inhibitory cells in the substantia gelatinosa shut the gate and pain impulses carried by small fibers can't proceed. (Some research suggests that large-fiber activity also inhibits small-fiber response to stimuli.)

• When small-fiber impulses predominate, T cells are activated and the pain message ascends to the brain. Apparently, T cells must receive a certain level of small-fiber stimulation before they become active. T-cell activity is influenced by the number of fibers carrying impulses, the fibers' firing rates, the balance of large- and small-fiber activity, and the activity of higher CNS structures.

• If pain impulses ascend to the brain, higher CNS structures—including the brain stem, thalamus, and cerebral cortex—can modulate pain by influencing T-cell activity. These structures control such factors as attention, emotion, and memory—thus helping to determine an individual's unique perception of pain.

Implications. The gate control theory explains why rubbing or massaging a sore spot immediately after an injury may relieve pain—the resulting large-fiber activity helps diminish the influence of small, pain-carrying fibers.

We've already discussed how release of endorphins and other endogenous opioids may explain the success of acupuncture and TENS. The gate control theory provides another possible explanation: cutaneous electrical activity stimulates large-diameter fibers, closing the gate to T-cell activation by small-diameter fibers.

How gate control modifies pain transmission

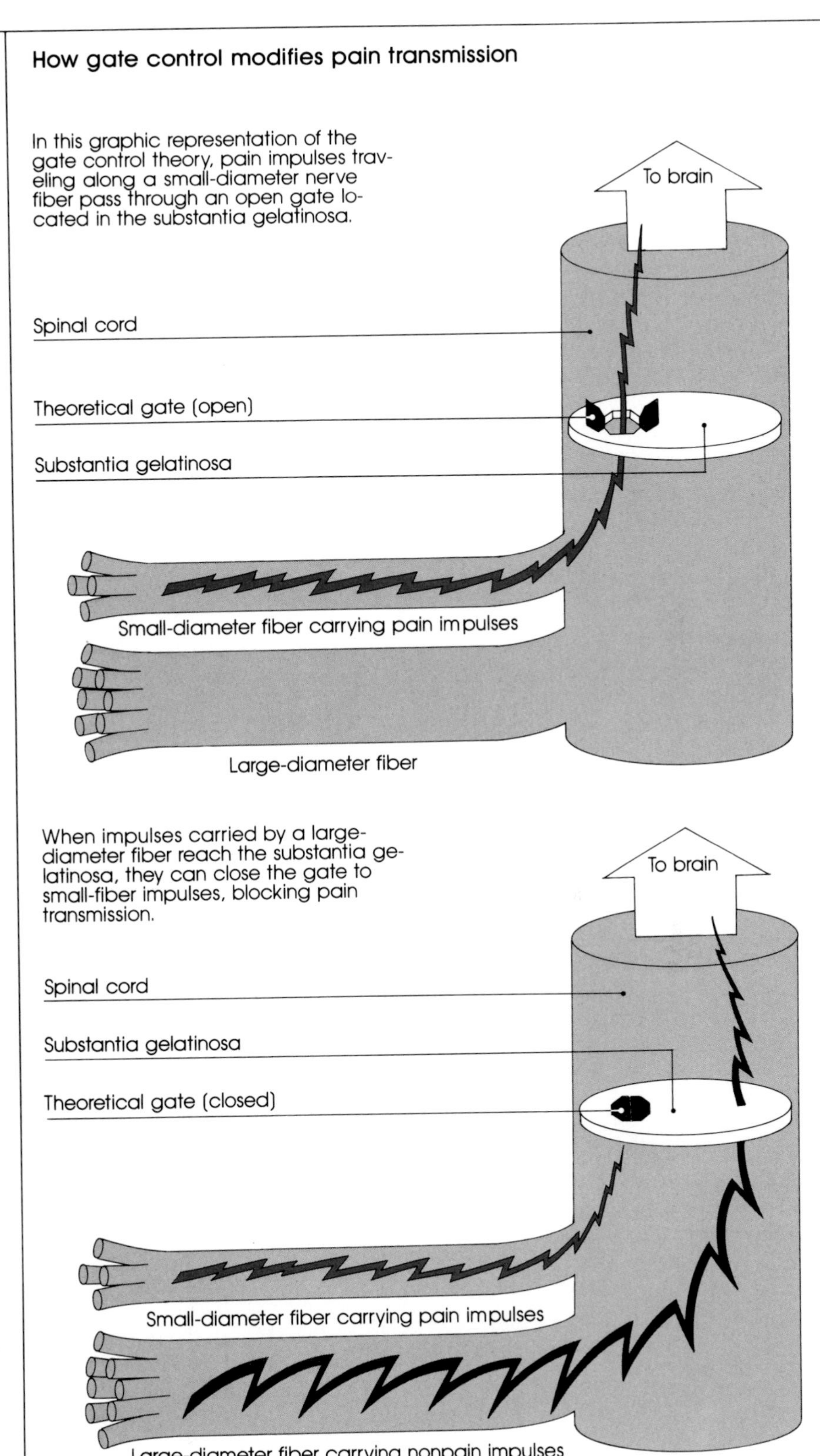

PAIN RESPONSES

REFERRED PAIN

Every nurse knows this classic symptom of myocardial infarction: pain radiating from the chest to the left arm and jaw. It's only one example of the referred pain phenomenon—pain that's felt away from the source of disease or injury. This type of pain is typically referred from visceral and deep somatic (nonvisceral) tissue.

Characteristics. Referred visceral pain usually corresponds to known dermatomes. In other words, the diseased or injured tissue and the reference tissue are supplied by the same spinal root. This may explain why referred pain occurs in predictable patterns. These patterns, along with other physical assessment findings, can have significant diagnostic value.

The pain of myocardial infarction isn't the only example of referred pain. Gallbladder pain, for instance, may be referred from the upper abdomen to the right shoulder tip. Why? Because the gallbladder lies adjacent to the right diaphragm, which is innervated by the third, fourth, and fifth cranial roots. These roots, which also innervate the right shoulder, refer the pain of gallbladder inflammation to this area. For similar reasons, spleen pain may be referred to the left shoulder; kidney pain to the flank or abdomen; and pain caused by a large abdominal aortic aneurysm to the lower back.

Although several possible explanations for referred pain exist, most authorities believe that it arises from CNS confusion at the spinal cord level, as explained by the *convergence theory*. Because visceral and somatic afferent fibers converge at the dorsal horn, the CNS misinterprets the visceral impulses as being somatic in origin.

Trigger points. Referred pain can be associated with a specific trigger point or area—a cutaneous spot that causes pain after even light stimulation. Well-known trigger areas for patients with heart disease include points along the chest and upper back. Firm pressure at one of these points (which are often associated with musculoskeletal pain) can produce sharp, stabbing, long-lasting pain. Interestingly, traditional acupuncture sites correspond well to these and other known trigger points.

Common referred pain sites

These anterior and posterior views of the body show where a patient might feel pain referred from various visceral organs.

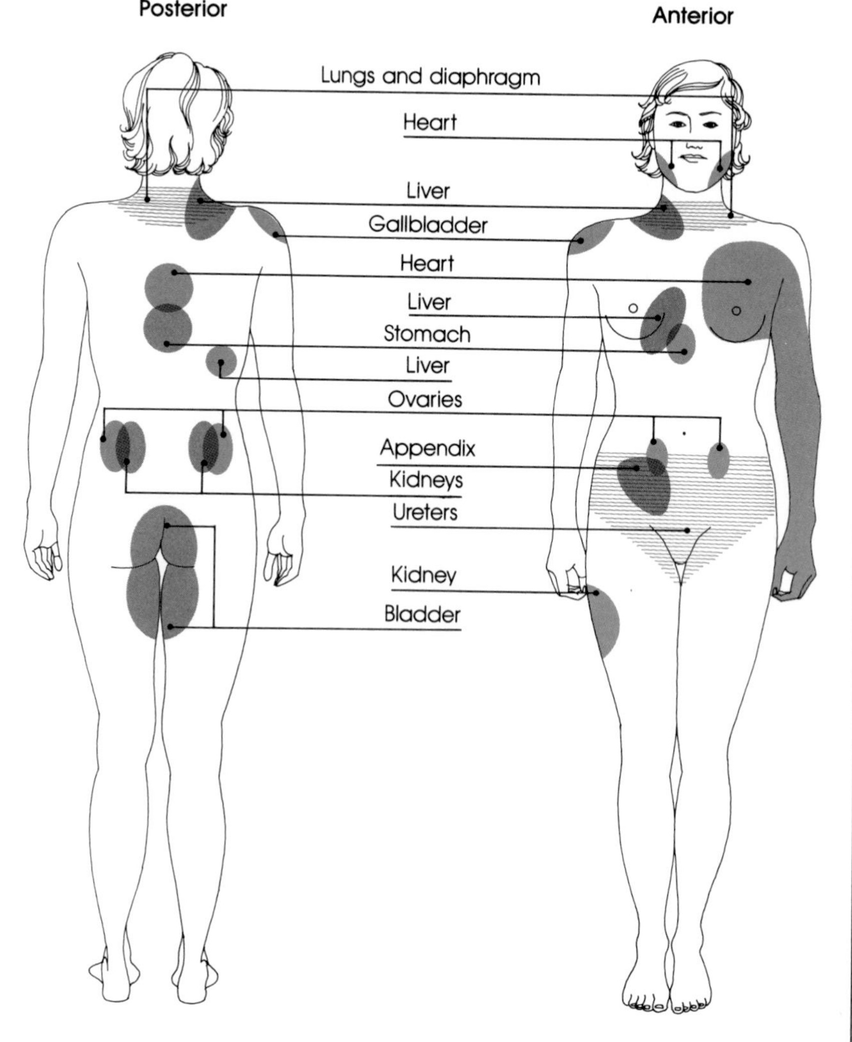

PSYCHOSOCIAL FACTORS

THREE-STAGED RESPONSE

When the central nervous system perceives pain, it prepares the body to respond. We classify pain response into three stages.

Activation. Also known as the *fight-or-flight* reaction, this stage begins immediately after pain stimulation. To prepare a person for defense or escape, the sympathetic nervous system initiates these responses:

- increased heart rate, cardiac contractility, and blood pressure, to boost cardiac output
- increased respiratory rate
- bronchiolar dilation, to improve alveolar ventilation
- blood flow diversion from peripheral tissues and the GI tract (causing nausea and a hollow feeling in the stomach), to improve blood supply to organs
- conversion of stored glycogen into glucose by the liver, to provide fuel and extra energy
- release of red blood cells from the spleen, to improve the blood's oxygen-carrying capacity
- pupil dilation.

Rebound. When pain's intense but brief, the parasympathetic nervous system takes over. Its effects are opposite to those of the sympathetic nervous system: respiratory rate, heart rate, and blood pressure drop.

Adaption. Following prolonged sympathetic stimulation (as in repetitive or chronic pain), the body no longer exhibits extreme sympathetic responses. In fact, most physiologic indicators (such as heart rate and blood pressure) are normal. As a result, you could conclude that his pain is negligible. Don't make this mistake. He could be experiencing severe, prolonged pain. The contrast between the chronic pain experience and the relative absence of sympathetic responses is one reason chronic pain is hard to recognize and treat.

THE PSYCHOLOGY OF PAIN

Although gate control and other pain theories attempt to explain the physiologic complexities of pain, all fall short of fully defining the pain phenomenon. The reason: No pain, from the slightest to the most severe, is purely organic. Rather, every pain is a combination of a physical sensation and an emotional response.

In the past, the emotional or psychological component of pain was usually overlooked or misinterpreted. A patient who complained frequently about pain was likely to be labeled a nuisance or a whiner who simply wanted attention. In contrast, a patient who never complained about pain (or who did so only occasionally) was assumed to be pain-free or to have only minor pain. In reality, both patients may have been experiencing severe pain. But because of stereotyped notions and misconceptions about pain, neither of them may have received adequate pain relief.

To avoid false assumptions and ineffective nursing measures, remember that all patients react differently to pain because of the psychological, social, and cultural influences that make them individuals. And these psychological factors—worry, anxiety, depression, fear—can intensify pain.

Consequently, to care effectively for a patient in pain, you must evaluate the psychosocial influences that help determine how he responds to and copes with pain. To do that, stay alert to the clues the patient reveals about himself: his emotions, values, attitudes, beliefs, and previous pain experiences. Then use this information, along with other assessment findings, to develop an appropriate nursing care plan.

PAIN AND PERSONALITY

Every patient's personality influences how he reacts to pain. Some patients' behavior accurately reflects the pain they feel. But in other patients, behavior exaggerates or masks what they're experiencing. To effectively evaluate and manage a patient's pain, familiarize yourself with each personality type discussed below. Then adjust your interventions appropriately.

- *An augmenter* amplifies pain sensation by focusing on it. He reacts with alarm and anxiety to each painful episode and may even lose his ability to function normally while he's having pain. He may also be reluctant to give up his symptoms. To determine the effectiveness of your intervention, observe his activity level following treatment. Don't rely on his verbal responses alone.
- *A minimizer* ignores or represses his pain. He may delay reporting symptoms, deny illness, and fail to adhere to medical regimens. Don't wait for this patient to ask for pain relief. Instead, ask him at regular intervals about his discomfort and offer some intervention.
- *An introvert* won't volunteer information about his pain. When asked, he answers tersely. Encourage him to talk about his pain by demonstrating sincere concern.
- *An extrovert* readily and openly describes his pain. But don't assume that he'll volunteer all the information. Assess him as thoroughly as your other patients, and document his responses.
- *A neurotic* patient is anxious, emotionally labile, and highly sensitive to pain, often complaining openly of even minor discomfort. Never ignore the patient's complaints or make light of them because of his behavior. Take care to intervene as quickly for him as you would for any patient.

PSYCHOSOCIAL FACTORS CONTINUED

PAIN AS A PSYCHIATRIC SYMPTOM

Pain can be the chief presenting complaint of a number of psychiatric disorders, including hysterical or conversion pain, schizophrenia, psychoses and dementias, malingering, hypochondriasis, and depression. The emotions that accompany these disorders—anxiety, depression, anger, guilt—often manifest themselves as pain.

Consequently, if the doctor has determined that the underlying cause of the patient's pain is psychiatric, you can relieve the patient's pain by treating his psychiatric disorder.

Remember, however, that pain can *cause* a psychiatric condition such as depression. A patient with chronic pain may become severely depressed by his persistent pain—possibly to the point of contemplating suicide. Continually assess such a patient's suicide risk. For example, you can ask him if he's ever felt so depressed that he wanted to die. If he has, ask if he has any plans for hurting himself now or later if the pain doesn't get better.

If your patient is potentially suicidal, immediately alert his doctor. Initiate suicide precautions, if appropriate.

HOW YOUR PATIENT INTERPRETS PAIN

How your patient reacts to pain depends in large part on two considerations: what the pain means to him and his previous pain experiences. By definition, pain is an unpleasant sensation. Paradoxically, however, a patient may accept pain, depending on circumstances and his interpretation of its significance.

Sometimes a necessary evil. A patient experiencing an acutely painful condition may withstand the pain surprisingly well if he associates it with a benefit. An athlete who's undergone successful orthopedic surgery to prolong his career, a woman giving birth to a healthy child, a patient recovering from cosmetic plastic surgery—all of these people are likely to tolerate pain well because they associate it with a positive outcome.

A classic example of the influence of pain interpretation on pain tolerance is H.K. Beecher's study of soldiers severely wounded in battle. Despite their injuries, most of the soldiers studied acknowledged little or no pain and didn't want pain medication. In contrast, Beecher found that civilian patients with similar surgical wounds required narcotics for relief. Beecher's conclusion? Because the soldiers' wounds removed them from battle and would probably lead to discharge, the pain represented a positive outcome. The civilian patients, on the other hand, could make no such positive association between acute pain and a future benefit. For them, fear and depression probably increased the pain they felt.

Physical surroundings can influence pain response. In a social setting, for example, a person who experiences unexpected pain may downplay his response. But in a hospital, where expressing pain is more acceptable, he might respond more openly.

Meaningless pain. A patient with chronic pain is likely to have a much different response to his condition. Because continuous or recurring pain serves no useful purpose—and because it's unrelenting—he can attach no positive significance to it. Instead, he perceives it as a threat to his body image and life-style—and possibly as a reminder of impending death.

Research refutes the common belief that chronic pain patients become more tolerant of pain as time passes. In fact, their suffering may intensify as anxiety, depression, and despair increase.

Prior experiences. Regardless of whether your patient suffers from chronic or acute pain, consider his previous pain experiences when planning his care.

Adults who experienced pain as children—either personally or by being exposed to the suffering of a family member or close friend—are more threatened by anticipated pain than adults without prior pain experience. As a result, they may be more sensitive to pain than other patients.

Similarly, past experiences with pain-relief interventions influence a patient's expectations for relief. For example, if he's tried a variety of pain-relief measures without success, he may have little hope that your interventions will help him.

SOCIOCULTURAL CONSIDERATIONS

Social and cultural differences may also affect a patient's pain response by influencing how he interprets pain and responds emotionally. Through an integration of cultural influences, social customs, and familial values and attitudes, the patient learns what kind of pain responses are appropriate within his sociocultural group.

Cultural considerations. Appropriate pain responses vary according to the individual's age and sex. In most cultures, for example, girls are more free to openly express pain than boys. Similarly, adults are expected to bear pain more stoically than children. Cultural standards also teach an individual:
- how much pain to tolerate
- what types of pain to report or complain about
- who to report pain to
- what type of treatment to seek.

Familial influences. While a patient's culture establishes overall standards for behavior, his family establishes values by emphasizing or deemphasizing various cultural and social standards. Learning begins early in childhood when pain behavior is rewarded, punished, or ignored. From one generation to the next, the family passes on specific beliefs, traditions, and customs that help determine how its members react under various circumstances.

Of course, family influences change as a child matures. By the time he's reached adulthood and has established his own identity and life-style, he may have modified and even rejected many of his family's values or taken on the values of another subgroup. If the patient's values conflict with his family's, he may feel additional stress and anxiety, particularly when his family is present. This may explain why patients act differently when family members visit. To care for the patient effectively, be aware of the influence the family may have on his attitudes and behavior toward pain and illness.

Avoid stereotyping. If you're familiar with accepted behavior within your patient's sociocultural or familial group, you can assess his pain responses (or lack of them) with greater insight. At the same time, however, you must remember that each patient is an individual, not a stereotype. Contrary to popular belief, not all Jewish and Italian-American patients are highly emotional; Irish Americans don't always deny pain; and Americans of Anglo-Saxon origins aren't always stoic. Despite cultural influences, each patient is unique—and so is his response to pain.

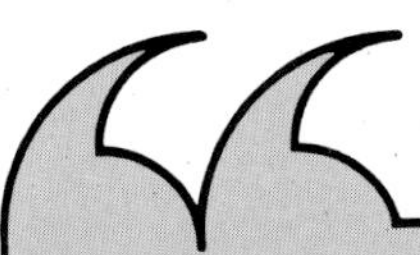

"The words a patient uses to report the emotions and physical sensations associated with pain are influenced by his ethnicity and language. So don't be too quick to assume that you understand what he's trying to say—especially if his native language and ethnic background differ from yours."

Marcia Luna, RN, MN, CS
Mental Health Clinical Nurse Specialist
UCLA Medical Center
Los Angeles

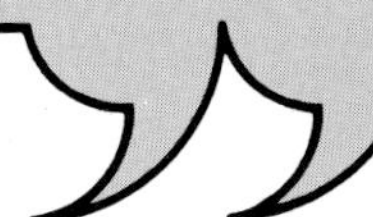

OTHER INFLUENCES ON PAIN RESPONSE

Besides cultural and familial influences, these factors influence a patient's pain response:
- *Body part involved.* In almost every culture, people learn not to show, touch, or discuss such body parts as the rectum and genitals. So when one of these body parts becomes painful, a patient may have difficulty talking about his pain.

  You can help him by broaching the subject in a nonthreatening way. For example, you might suggest that he write down his feelings about it. Or give him a diagram or sketch to refer to. A simple pain scale may also help him describe his pain.
- *Socioeconomic status.* Research indicates that patients with higher incomes have more pain tolerance than those with lower incomes. One reason may be that a patient who's financially secure views pain and illness more as a temporary inconvenience than as a possible disruption of his life and livelihood. This patient probably has more job security, better health insurance coverage, and easier access to appropriate health care. For all these reasons, he's less threatened by pain and illness than a person with a lower income.
- *Religious beliefs.* Because a person's religious convictions affect how he views himself, they also influence how he responds to pain. If religion is a source of strength for him, he may be comforted by praying for relief. Or his religion may provide a reason for his suffering, making the pain easier to accept. Another patient might regard pain as a punishment that he must endure or seek forgiveness for.
- *Belief in folk medicine.* Many patients follow the advice of nonprofessionals—neighbors, rela-

CONTINUED ON PAGE 22

PSYCHOSOCIAL FACTORS CONTINUED

OTHER INFLUENCES ON PAIN RESPONSE
CONTINUED

tives, and friends—to treat illness. Folk remedies range from eating or drinking herbal preparations to wearing copper bracelets or other ornaments to ward off evil spirits. Unfortunately, many patients seek medical help only after such remedies have failed and their condition has become an emergency.

To care effectively for a patient who relies on folk medicine, first find out if he distrusts established medicine. If he does, he may deny his pain or fail to report it in an attempt to avoid your intervention. To help this patient better accept hospital care and respond more openly and honestly to your questions about his pain, find out what nontraditional therapies he's been using. Then, try to combine these nontraditional practices with his prescribed medical regimen (provided, of course, that they don't interfere with legitimate medical and nursing care). For example, a patient could wear a copper bracelet or use an herbal ointment while also taking prescribed pain medications.

• *Language.* A patient's vocabulary affects how he perceives pain, what pain means to him, and how he describes it. The English language, for example, is rich in words that emphasize the physical aspect of pain or refer to danger or harm. Consequently, English-speaking patients usually express even emotional distress in terms of physical pain. Conversely, the Japanese language has no special terms that easily describe the physical qualities of pain. As a result, the Japanese usually describe their pain in psychological, rather than physical, terms.

CRITICAL QUESTIONS

ASSESSING SOCIOCULTURAL INFLUENCES

To better meet the pain sufferer's needs, find out how his sociocultural background has shaped his responses to pain by asking the following questions:

• Where were your parents or ancestors born? How long has your family lived in this country? Do you speak a second language at home? If so, what?
• Do you still hold to the values and customs of your ethnic group? If not, what changes have you made?
• Where do you live?
• Has the pain affected your work or life-style?
• How is your pain affecting your family? Is it bringing them closer together, causing problems, or having no effect?
• Did you treat your illness at home? If so, how?
• Did you seek treatment from anyone other than a health professional before coming here? Who was he, and what did he do?
• Do you use any home remedies? Describe them.
• What's your religion? Do you have any religious beliefs about treating illness?
• Have you ever tried faith healing?
• How do you view your illness in general? Do you feel you're in control of it?
• What do you think caused your pain?
• What do you fear most about your pain? How do you expect treatment to help you?

As you review and analyze the patient's responses, ask yourself the following questions. Your answers will help you develop an appropriate care plan.

• Is the patient concerned about the pain itself or its implications?
• Does he want to be asked about his pain? Or would he prefer not to be reminded of it?
• During a painful episode, does he prefer to be alone so he can cope with the pain himself? Or does he prefer to be alone for fear of responding emotionally to his pain in your presence?
• Does he want visitors to share his pain? Or does he view them as a distraction from his pain?
• Do his relationships with family and friends affect his pain? If so, how?
• Does he believe drugs are unnatural pain-relief measures? Does he fear becoming addicted to them?
• Does he expect immediate relief from your interventions?
• Does he trust you and other staff members?

EXPLORING YOUR PAIN ATTITUDES

Do you have a preconceived notion about how a patient should respond to pain? If so, how do you react when a patient fails to meet your expectations? If you consider him childish or merely an attention-seeker, you may be unable to assess his pain accurately or devise an effective nursing care plan for him.

Occasionally, you'll have conflicts between your own expectations and a patient's responses. But don't let your values interfere with the professional nursing care he's entitled to. By being aware of the following prejudices and myths about pain and pain responses, you'll be more sensitive to your patient's needs.

Professional prejudices. Studies indicate that health-care professionals tend to infer less pain than a patient actually experiences. In fact, those who have the closest physical contact with a pain sufferer are most likely to minimize his pain. Why? Possibly health professionals try to protect themselves emotionally by denying that the patient is really suffering. Or, after frequent exposure to people in pain, they may simply view it as routine and ordinary.

Another factor that may influence how you view your patient's pain is the medical and nursing professions' emphasis on physical assessment findings rather than the patient's subjective report. In nursing school and on the job, you may have learned to respond to pain only if the patient has a proven organic problem.

In many instances, however, pain produces few physical signs and symptoms. Of course, during an acute pain episode you may see signs of autonomic nervous system response; for example, pulse or blood pressure changes. But with a chronic pain patient, you won't see physiologic changes. Consequently, the patient's subjective response to pain is about all you have to go on. Try to understand what your patient is experiencing from his viewpoint. If you can't, or if you begin to feel disdain or dislike for the patient because of his pain-related behavior, talk to your supervisor or colleagues about it. To establish an objective and therapeutic relationship with any patient, you must put aside your own personal values and concentrate on the patient's.

No pain is routine or ordinary to the patient experiencing it. When pain occurs, he needs help and he needs you to believe him.

Pain myths. Despite increased knowledge about pain and the various methods of relieving it, a number of misconceptions still exist. Read about some of the most common myths below. If you're still holding on to some of them, start working now to dispel them.

• *Pain caused by emotional responses—fear, worry, depression—doesn't require treatment.* As we mentioned earlier, all pain has a psychological and a physiologic component. Regardless of the cause, the pain sufferer requires your attention and proper intervention. Frequently assure the patient that you believe his pain is real and that you'll work with him to try to relieve it.

• *You can distinguish the real pain sufferer from the faker.* Too often nurses feel that unless a patient looks like he's in pain, he's not really suffering and doesn't require intervention. But every patient responds to pain differently. And since only the patient knows what he's feeling, believe him when he says he has pain and try to relieve it.

Refusing to believe that a patient has pain or withholding medication and other pain-relief measures because you think he's a malingerer or drug-seeker only leads to more problems. If the patient does have psychiatric or drug-related problems, involve the entire health-care team—including a mental health professional—in the assessment and management of his condition.

• *Placebos can help you distinguish the faker from the true pain sufferer.* Placebos can, in fact, provide effective pain relief for about one in three patients. Although the exact mechanism is unknown, the placebo response may be associated with endorphin release. Don't assume, therefore, that a patient who responds to a placebo is a faker or a malingerer. (For details on endorphins and other endogenous opioids, review pages 14 to 15.)

"Don't assume that placebos relieve only psychogenic—not physical—pain. For over 25 years, double-blind studies have shown that cancer and postoperative patients get pain relief from placebos at least one third of the time—and these patients have pain that's clearly physical in origin."

Margo McCaffery, RN, MS, FAAN
Consultant in the Nursing Care of People with Pain
Santa Monica, Calif.

PSYCHOSOCIAL FACTORS CONTINUED

CHRONIC PAIN: THE ROAD TO ACCEPTANCE

Dealing with a chronic pain sufferer can be overwhelming. While acute pain—for example, after surgery—can be excruciating, healing usually brings permanent relief. But dealing with chronic pain becomes a new way of life. Not only does chronic pain change a patient's body image, it may impede his ability to walk, talk, sleep, or eat. It may also impede his ability to function professionally, socially, and even sexually. Many chronic pain sufferers undergo complete personality changes and isolate themselves from family and friends.

With your help, the chronic pain sufferer can learn to cope. The first step is to develop a program of effective pain-relief measures. The second is to help him adjust his life-style to accommodate the pain.

But coming to terms with chronic pain isn't easy. Most patients pass through a series of emotional stages before learning how to cope effectively. Some vascillate between stages; others get mired in a particular one. To keep the chronic pain sufferer moving in the right direction, familiarize yourself with the following stages. Then, accept and support the patient throughout each one.

- *Denial.* The patient refuses to believe that his pain can't be diagnosed or cured.
- *Anger or depression.* The patient stops trying to cope and becomes dependent on others.
- *Defiance.* The patient will do anything to get pain relief but refuses to change his life-style because of the pain.
- *Withdrawal.* The patient refuses most pain-relief measures and makes every effort to maintain his normal life-style.
- *Seeking help.* The patient makes efforts to get relief from his pain and is willing to adjust his life-style to accommodate his pain.
- *Coping.* The patient uses effective pain-relief strategies and resumes normal activities only when he can do them safely and without increasing his pain.

HELPING THE PATIENT COPE: YOUR ROLE

The first step toward helping a pain sufferer is to *believe* him when he says he has pain. Because pain is subjective, the only person who can judge it accurately is the patient himself. He's the ultimate authority on his pain. Once you acknowledge him as such, you can begin helping him use his own strengths to cope with his pain.

How? First, remember that many pain sufferers function best in a quiet, soothing environment. Try to eliminate or minimize such noxious stimuli as bright lights or a loud television or radio (unless the television or radio helps distract him from his pain). To help decrease the patient's anxiety between painful episodes, give him access to the sun room, cafeteria, or chapel. And, if possible, establish a support system for him with a chaplain, social worker, or other qualified person. Talking about his pain experience with trained personnel helps the patient clarify any misconceptions he has about his pain. Regularly scheduled visits from family and friends also give the patient something to look forward to and help him pass the time.

Sensitivity to your patient's pain experience is only the first step. But it's the foundation for all your nursing interventions, from giving medications to providing comfort measures to patient teaching.

One pain control aid: A quiet environment

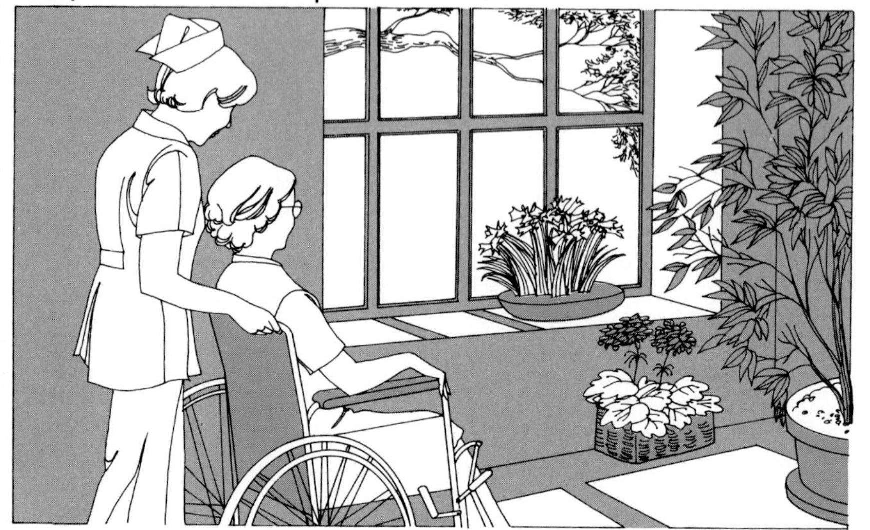

ASSESSMENT

IRST STEPS
ISTORY
OCUMENTATION
ARE PLANS

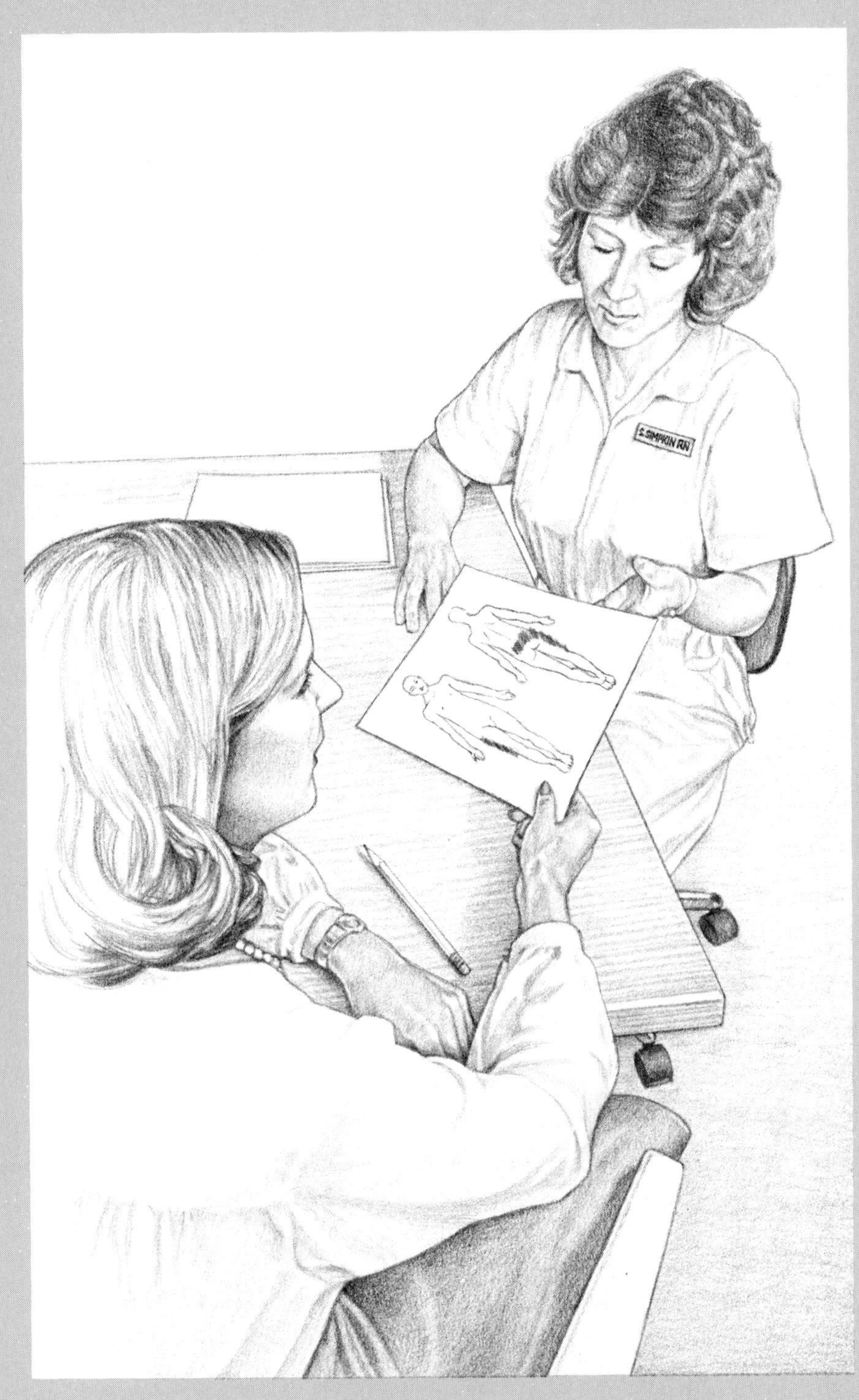

FIRST STEPS

PAIN ASSESSMENT: PRELIMINARY CONSIDERATIONS

In years past, most nurses believed a patient's pain was one thing and managing it was another. Nurses had little—if anything—to do with the systematic assessment of pain and were responsible only for administering pain medication as ordered.

Today, of course, you're responsible for far more than just dispensing medication. You're also responsible for assessing your patient's pain and implementing a nursing care plan especially designed for his needs.

But accurately assessing pain isn't as easy as it sounds. While the pain of a patient recovering from abdominal surgery is obvious and expected, another patient's chronic pain may be less obvious and easily overlooked. Yet both patients need your intervention.

Because each patient's pain response is unique, your assessment of how he perceives his pain must be the foundation of his care plan. You also need to know whether his pain is chronic or acute, since appropriate intervention hinges on this finding.

Another part of pain assessment is evaluating the factors that alleviate or exacerbate your patient's pain. By continually reassessing the duration, intensity, and type of pain your patient's experiencing, you can gauge the effectiveness of your interventions.

Key questions. Make pain evaluation a part of the assessment process for every patient—regardless of whether pain is his presenting problem. Your general nursing assessment form should contain a few questions such as these:

- Are you experiencing any pain? If so, how would you describe it?
- How have you managed pain in the past?
- What type of medication do you usually take for pain—for example, a headache? Does this usually provide you with relief?

Pain assessment. If your initial assessment indicates that your patient's in pain, your next step is to gather as much information as possible about his condition. In this section, we'll discuss assessment tools and methods that can help you do so. Your ultimate goal, of course, is to formulate a nursing diagnosis and care plan that will enable you to provide quality care for him.

To avoid missing any important pieces of the pain puzzle, adopt a systematic approach. The SOAPIE format, which provides a handy framework for both assessment and subsequent intervention, covers these areas:

- subjective data
- objective data
- assessment (ongoing)
- plan of intervention
- intervention and implementation
- evaluation of the implemented plan.

With this detailed approach, you can initiate nursing measures that are appropriate for your patient and his specific pain problems.

A word of caution. When evaluating pain—or responses to pain-relief measures—don't make the mistake of comparing one patient to another. Remember, each person's pain experience is unique. The only valid comparison you can make is between the patient's past and current conditions. Your initial assessment provides a record of your patient's condition before intervention; use it to evaluate the success of your nursing care plan. And remember, your patient's the best judge of his pain relief. Make sure you ask him for his opinions on the success of the interventions.

Pain assessment: The decision process

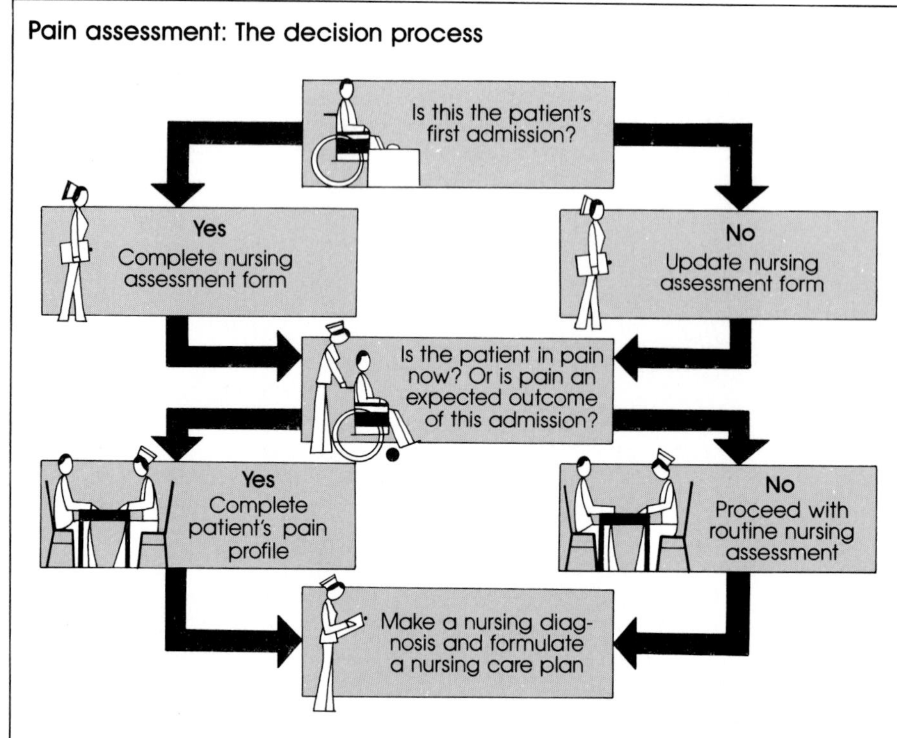

YOUR ROLE

As a nurse, you spend more time with your patient than with any other member of the health-care team. That's why your part in the pain assessment process is so critical. By gathering, documenting, and evaluating data about your patient's pain, you can effectively intervene and help to control his pain.

To do so, you must:

• recognize that pain assessment is a joint process requiring input from the patient and close family members or friends
• know your patient's pain and medical history
• choose an appropriate assessment tool for your patient, and incorporate its use into your ongoing assessment
• know what pain patterns are associated with specific conditions, such as acute myocardial infarction
• formulate appropriate nursing diagnoses
• incorporate your nursing diagnoses into the total care plan
• follow a multidisciplinary health team approach when coordinating pain-management efforts
• provide an avenue for ongoing feedback and assessment of your patient's needs through staff meetings and complete, ongoing documentation
• be sensitive to your patient's possible reluctance to modify his behavior as a part of pain control
• watch for potential problems that may prevent you from effectively managing your patient's pain-control needs: inadequate staffing; differing philosophies among health team members regarding pain management and medication administration; your own biases; and poor communication among health team members, the patient, and his family.

Using body diagrams to depict pain

By graphically representing his pain, your patient can help you understand what he feels. A patient with chronic lower back pain and an ulcer might mark these body diagrams as shown.

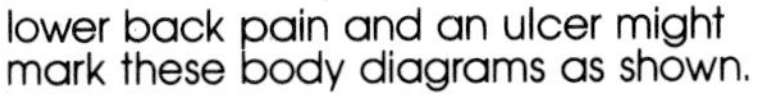

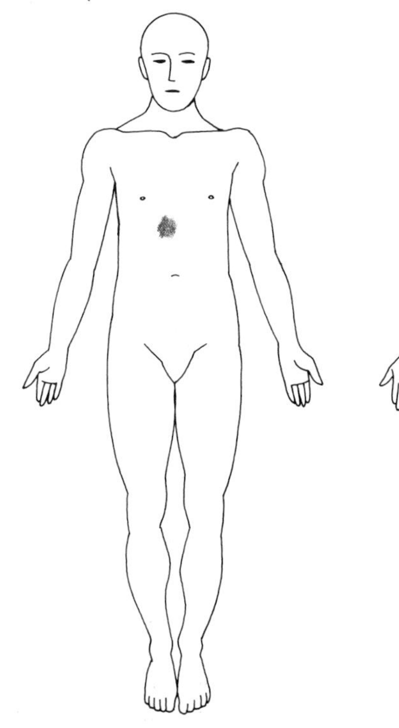

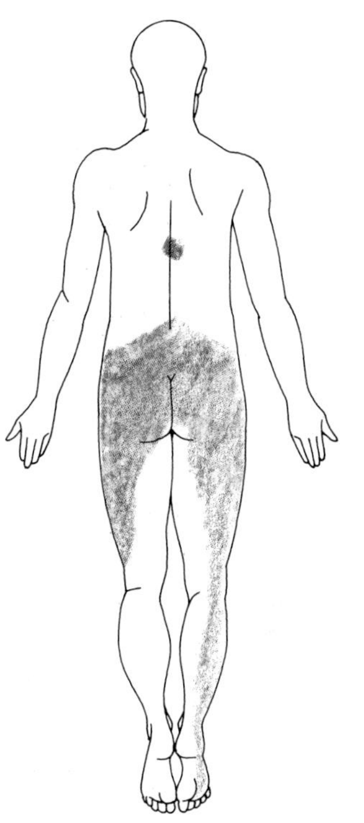

PAIN ASSESSMENT TIPS

On the following page, you'll find some suggested guidelines to follow during your assessment interview. In addition, make sure you explore these aspects of your patient's pain:

• *Onset and duration.* If his pain is episodic, find out if anything triggers its onset. For example, a patient with angina may begin to feel pain after an argument. Also, find out if he recognizes any pattern to his pain; for example, if it's more severe at certain times of the day.
• *Location.* Provide your patient with body diagrams like those shown above, and ask him to mark the painful areas. Also have him point to the painful areas on his own body. If his pain radiates, ask him to indicate its most severe point and to trace its pathway outward. *Important:* No matter how much you know about your patient's condition, don't make assumptions about the location of his pain. If he's recovering from abdominal surgery, for example, you expect him to have abdominal pain. But don't assume that's the only pain he's having. By failing to inquire further, you might miss signs of a complication, such as acute myocardial infarction or wound dehiscence.
• *Quality.* Ask your patient to describe his pain. Avoid such leading questions as "Is the pain throbbing?" Instead, use an open-ended statement like: "Tell me what your pain feels like." Carefully note and document your patient's exact words. His

CONTINUED ON PAGE 28

FIRST STEPS CONTINUED

PAIN ASSESSMENT TIPS
CONTINUED

reply may help you determine if his pain's superficial (a sharp, well-localized feeling) or visceral (dull and poorly localized). His description may also give you a clue to the condition causing the pain; for example, patients typically describe the pain of myocardial infarction as viselike, crushing, suffocating, heavy, or constricting. Similarly, patients with ulcers may describe their pain as burning or gnawing.

• *Intensity.* To help you determine whether your patient's pain is mild, moderate, severe, or overwhelming, ask him to rate its intensity on a scale of 1 to 10 (with 1 representing the least intense pain level). In addition to being easy to document, this assessment method helps you evaluate your nursing interventions. (See page 33 for an example of a linear scale.)

• *Aggravating and mitigating factors.* Position changes and bodily functions such as defecation and micturition can aggravate some kinds of pain; with other kinds, such factors have little or no effect. Likewise, such coping techniques as relaxation and distraction can relieve some types of pain. By knowing what's likely to increase or decrease your patient's pain, you can devise a more effective care plan.

• *Associated signs.* Finally, assess your patient for such signs and symptoms as blood pressure changes, tachycardia, skin color changes, diminished pulses, diaphoresis, and hyperventilation. Also observe for facial expressions and gestures that reflect pain, discomfort, or anxiety. Although your patient is the best authority on his own pain, your observations and other findings provide valuable insight into his condition and how he copes with it.

GUIDELINES FOR PAIN ASSESSMENT

Tailor your pain assessment to the patient's specific complaint and the pain's location. Although all of the following points won't be relevant to every patient's condition, you can adapt them as necessary.

HEAD PAIN (HEADACHES)

Ask about:
• visual disturbances
• dizziness
• vertigo
• nosebleeds
• ringing in ears
• muscle weakness
• seizures
• head injuries or recent trauma

Observe/inspect for:
• discharge from ears or nose
• breath odors
• abnormal gait or posture
• facial asymmetry
• enlarged lymph nodes
• edema

BREAST PAIN

Ask about:
• lumps or masses
• discharge from nipples

Observe/inspect for:
• asymmetry
• skin color changes
• discharge or bleeding from nipples
• breast engorgement

CHEST (RESPIRATORY) PAIN

Ask about:
• cough
• hemoptysis (color, frequency, and amount)
• shortness of breath (dyspnea)
• wheezing
• sputum (color, frequency, and amount)
• recent chest X-ray
• history of emphysema, asthma, bronchitis, pneumonia, or pleurisy
• recent trauma or injury

Observe/inspect for:
• chest asymmetry
• diaphoresis
• pursed lip breathing
• nostril flaring
• shortness of breath when speaking
• cyanosis
• finger clubbing
• extreme apprehension or agitation
• rapid, very deep, very shallow, or depressed respirations
• posterior or anterior chest wounds, lesions, masses, scars, or rib deformities
• use of accessory muscles
• barrel chest

CHEST (CARDIOVASCULAR) PAIN

Ask about:
• shortness of breath
• fatigue and weakness
• palpitations
• light-headedness, lapses of consciousness
• cardiac history

Observe/inspect for:
• dyspnea
• diaphoresis
• ankle edema
• cyanosis
• neck vein distention
• change in heart rate or rhythm
• abdominal pulsations
• heaves or lifts in anterior chest (visible heartbeat)

STOMACH (GASTROINTESTINAL) PAIN

Ask about:
• changes in eating or bowel habits
• anorexia
• nausea
• vomiting (frequency, color, and amount)
• diarrhea (frequency, consis-

tency, and amount)
- constipation
- belching or passing gas
- weight loss
- hemorrhoids

Observe/inspect for:
- shiny skin over abdomen
- distention
- jaundice
- pruritus
- blood in stool
- lumps or masses
- ascites

URINARY (GENITOURINARY) PAIN

Ask about:
- urinary frequency, urgency, or hesitancy
- urine color changes
- urinary output changes (more, less, or none at all)
- history of kidney stones or urinary problems
- blood in urine

Observe/inspect for:
- amount, color, and character of urine
- inflammation or discharge in genital area
- bladder distention
- kidney enlargement
- incontinence

LOWER ABDOMINAL (GYNECOLOGIC) PAIN

Ask about:
- menstrual periods (duration, flow, cycle regularity, and date of last menses), bleeding between periods (metrorrhagia), or excess bleeding during menses (menorrhagia)
- pregnancies (gravida or para)
- cramps
- menopause
- discharge
- lesions
- abnormal bleeding
- pruritus

Observe/inspect for:
- discharge
- lesions
- mass (exerting pressure on surrounding tissues)
- overstretching of muscles, ligaments, and skin

EXTREMITY (MUSCULOSKELETAL) PAIN

Ask about:
- recent trauma or injury
- joint stiffness
- tenderness
- redness or swelling
- deformity
- limitation of movement
- numbness
- tingling
- difficulty walking
- intermittent claudication

Observe/inspect for:
- rashes
- color changes (cyanosis or jaundice)
- edema
- lacerations or bruises
- deformity
- pigmentation changes
- crepitus
- grip strength deficit

LOWER BACK (LUMBOSACRAL) PAIN

Ask about:
- trauma or injury (recent spinal trauma, heavy lifting, or back strain)
- voiding or defecating difficulties
- discomfort during coughing, sneezing, or straining
- buttock or leg pain
- exercise habits
- recent weight gain
- numbness, tingling, or prickling sensations

Observe/inspect for:
- abnormal gait or posture
- limited range of motion

KNOW YOUR BIASES

How do you feel about pain—and people in pain? Chances are, your attitudes vary according to the individual and the type of pain he's feeling.

Like all of us, you have beliefs and prejudices formed by a lifetime of experiences. But as a nurse, you can't allow your own prejudices to interfere with the pain-relief interventions each patient deserves.

Do you expect all patients in pain to display the same (or similar) signs and symptoms? If so, you may overlook the needs of a chronic pain patient who suffers in silence. Do you strongly disapprove of certain kinds of people, such as alcoholics or felons? If so, you may unconsciously make pain relief a lower priority for them than you would for other patients.

You may have heard co-workers—or even yourself—making statements like those below. Be aware that they reflect preconceptions based on:
- ethnic background ("The Chinese can tolerate more pain than Italians.")
- sex ("Women ask for pain medication at the drop of a hat.")
- age ("Geriatric patients are always complaining about something.")
- physical appearance ("If she weren't so fat, she wouldn't have fallen and broken her leg in the first place.")
- cause of pain ("An uncomplicated appendectomy isn't very painful.").

Of course, you can't deposit your emotions and values at the door when you arrive at work—nor should you. But you can be aware of your own prejudices and try to prevent them from compromising the quality nursing care you want to give every patient.

HISTORY

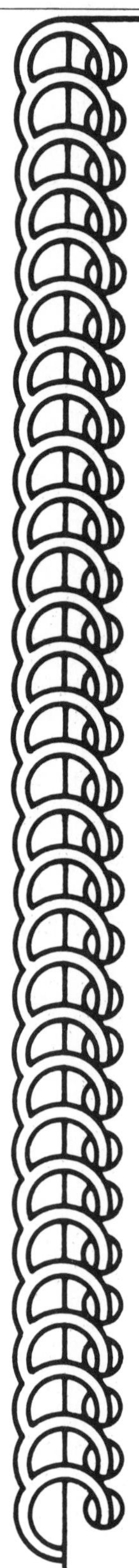

CRITICAL QUESTIONS

TAKING A PAIN HISTORY

When your patient's in pain, find out as much as possible about what he's feeling by asking him the right questions. Use this checklist as a guide.

During the interview, take care not to confuse your patient by using clinical terms. Document his responses in his own words; for example, "a tingling feeling" or "throbbing like a jackhammer." And remember, the success of your interview depends, in part, on the warmth and concern you convey to the patient. *Important:* If your patient denies being in pain, try using another word, such as *discomfort* or *pressure.*

Pain history

- What was the worst pain you ever experienced? What caused it? What relieved it?
- How long did this pain last?
- How would you describe it?

Medication history

- What drugs have you taken to relieve pain? Did they work? Did they cause any adverse effects? If so, what were they?
- Are you allergic or sensitive to any drugs? If so, which ones? What happens when you take them?

Present pain

- Are you presently in pain? Where is the pain located? Describe how it feels. How does this pain compare to the worst pain you've ever had?
- What relieves the pain—repositioning yourself, relaxing, or taking medication? Does anything (for example, eating) make your pain worse? Does body position, time of day, weather, or any specific activity affect your pain?
- Have you noticed any pattern in the way your pain comes and goes?
- Does the pain seem to be the same, or is it getting worse?
- Has the pain interfered with your day-to-day activities? How?
- Do you experience any other symptoms along with your pain (for example, blurred vision, rapid heartbeat, or shortness of breath)?
- How do you cope with the pain at home?
- Can you tell me any other details about you and your pain that health team members should know?

CHRONIC PAIN: SPECIAL CONSIDERATIONS

As part of your pain assessment, determine whether your patient is suffering chronic, rather than acute, pain. As we'll discuss later in this book, some interventions are more effective for chronic pain; others, for acute pain.

Acute versus chronic pain. By one practical definition, acute pain is temporary, lasting less than 6 months. Chronic pain, on the other hand, continues or recurs over a prolonged period—6 months or more. As a rule, acute pain is more easily managed than chronic pain.

In contrast, a patient with chronic pain may have little hope that the pain will *ever* subside. Chances are, earlier efforts to relieve the pain have failed, and he doubts that anyone can really help him. This patient's goals may be considerably different from those of a patient with acute pain.

Coping with chronic pain. Over time, a patient with chronic pain may develop extraordinary psychological coping mechanisms that permit him to continue functioning despite his handicap. These mechanisms, as valuable as they may be to him, can stand between you and a thorough pain assessemnt.

For example, your patient may be uncooperative or manipulative; because he can't control his pain, he may compensate by attempting to control his environment. Or he may be completely absorbed by his pain and unusually dependent on his family, friends, or you. Some patients may choose to remain in pain for personal reasons.

When caring for any chronic pain patient, you must be especially sensitive to the attitudes and concerns that shape his behavior. Because his perception of pain is so closely tied to his self-image and feelings of self-worth, he may be reluctant to discuss the subject honestly and openly. (This is particularly true if the pain involves a body part that he's embarrassed to talk about—for example, the rectum or the genitals).

Interview tips. Because your patient may be apprehensive or anxious about talking to you, plan to interview him in a private, relaxed setting. Explain how important an accurate pain assessment is for treatment. Using an informal manner, ask open-ended questions. Be a good listener, and encourage him to elaborate on his responses.

Keep in mind that your patient may have answered the same questions repeatedly. Try to avoid duplicating information that other health team members have already documented.

At right, you'll find a list of questions to guide you when assessing a patient with chronic pain. Use them to help you determine what significance the pain has for the patient. Does he accept his condition as permanent, or does he hope that drugs, surgery, or some other treatment will eventually eliminate it? Does he believe that pain devalues his worth as a person? Does he associate it with impending death? Perhaps he denies having pain altogether or chooses to ignore it. He may even feel that he somehow deserves to suffer. By gaining insight into his feelings about pain, you can design a nursing care plan that's appropriate for him. *Note:* Your patient's cultural, educational, and religious background influence his attitude toward pain. For a review of such psychosocial factors, see pages 19 to 24.

ASSESSING CHRONIC PAIN

When interviewing a chronic pain patient, you'll ask many of the same questions you'd pose during a general pain-assessment interview. But the questions below are particularly important.

Keep in mind that a patient with chronic pain probably has a long history, so be prepared to spend extra time with him. Check records from previous hospitalizations as well as the doctor's notes for additional information. Also, solicit information from the patient's family and friends; you'll need their help to intervene effectively.

- How long have you had this pain?
- Describe the pain. Did it develop quickly or slowly?
- Is the pain continuous, or does it sometimes go away? If it comes and goes, how long does it continue at one time?
- How would you compare this pain to pain you've had in the past?
- Do you take medication for the pain? If so, what? Does it relieve your pain?
- Have you tried any other pain-relief methods?
- Have you ever had surgery to try to relieve the pain? What type of surgery did you have? Did it help?
- How do you cope with this pain?
- What do you think caused it?
- How has it affected your life? Has it affected your relationships with others? If so, in what way?
- Do you work? Has your pain affected your ability to work?
- Have you ever gone to a pain clinic or attended a structured pain program?
- If so, briefly describe the program. Did it help? Are you currently attending this clinic? If not, why did you stop?
- How do you think we can help you?

Since many patients with chronic pain become depressed and potentially suicidal, be sure to assess your patient's suicide risk by asking the following questions:

- How do you feel about yourself? Do you ever feel so bad that you want to die? Do you feel that way now?

WHEN YOUR PATIENT HAS ACUTE PAIN

What do you do when a patient is in so much pain that you can't reasonably expect to take a complete and detailed history? Limit your questions to those most pertinent to his present pain. Likewise, limit your observation and inspection to those areas directly related to pain.

Consider, for example, Richard Paley—a 41-year-old steel salesman who's been admitted to your unit with acute abdominal pain. Because you observe that he's restless and having difficulty speaking, you'll want to phrase your questions so he can answer in as few words as possible.

You might ask:

- When did the pain start?
- What brought it on?
- Where is the pain located?
- Are you experiencing any other symptoms, such as nausea or vomiting?
- Have you ever had pain like this before? If so, tell me about it.

Ask him to rate his pain on a scale of 1 to 10, with 1 representing no pain and 10 the worst pain he's ever felt. This will help you evaluate the success of subsequent pain-relief measures. Also, observe him for nonverbal pain clues, such as grimacing and rigid body positioning. Document all your findings.

HISTORY CONTINUED

NONVERBAL PAIN CLUES

Your patient's behavior and appearance provide you with nonverbal clues about his pain. From the moment you meet, begin to watch for these clues. Your observations, along with a thorough patient history, give a more complete view of your patient's pain.

During assessment, be especially alert for discrepancies between how the patient describes his pain and what his behavior or appearance conveys. His nonverbal messages can provide valuable clues to how he really feels.

Your observations. In addition to such obvious signs of pain as crying, moaning, or screaming, consider the following clues potential expressions of pain:

- excessive demands, complaints, or appeals about trivial as well as important matters
- repetition of words
- grimacing, frowning, squinting
- tense facial muscles
- drawing arms or legs close to the body
- clutching or rubbing the painful area
- nervousness
- muscle guarding, unusual posture, or fetal position
- inactivity; lying very still in bed.

Note: Some patients—especially children—may respond to pain with *increased* activity.

Other indicators. Also watch for autonomic nervous system changes (more common with acute than chronic pain) and changes in the activities of daily living; for example:

- increased blood pressure
- increased pulse rate
- increased respiratory rate
- pupil dilation
- skin color changes (flushing or pallor)
- nausea, vomiting, and other GI changes
- diaphoresis
- altered sleep or rest patterns
- diminished ability to concentrate
- decreased social interactions (withdrawal from family or friends)

Looking inward. Your patient's not the only person communicating nonverbally. You are, too. To determine whether you unintentionally send your patient negative messages, ask yourself:

- Do my voice, word choices, posture, gestures, or facial expressions convey a message that will discourage a successful relationship with my patient?
- Do I avoid eye contact, shift my weight from side to side, glance at my watch, stare into space, or speak in a cool and uncaring tone of voice?
- Do I always appear rushed or hurried?

One of the best ways to send your patient a positive message is to sit down with him periodically and talk with him. Even 5 minutes of uninterrupted conversation tells him that you want to help. You may be surprised at how readily he relaxes his guard when he knows you care.

Special Note:

When you detect a discrepancy between a patient's verbal and nonverbal behavior—and you can't resolve the discrepancy by talking with the patient—consult family members. They may be able to contribute details he's reluctant to tell you.

SETTING PAIN-MANAGEMENT GOALS

During your assessment, make your patient feel more comfortable by learning about his concerns and needs. By doing so, you can help him set pain-management goals.

Appropriate goals vary from patient to patient, depending on each individual and the type of pain he's experiencing. A patient with chronic pain, for example, is likely to have goals that are far different from those of an acute pain sufferer. Use the information on the preceding pages to help you determine what goals are appropriate for your patient.

Don't forget, however, that your patient's preferences are essential for setting meaningful goals. Specifically ask him about his thoughts and feelings about his condition.

Because the patient's needs may not be what you expect, a simple question like "What can we do to help you?" may elicit surprising—and valuable—information.

Don't assume that your patient is pain-free just because he's taking medication or is undergoing special therapy (for example, with a TENS unit). Effective pain management takes time. A patient with pain—especially chronic pain—may need to identify his concerns and set realistic goals before he can fully manage his condition. For example, he may decide that "in 6 months, I'll be able to play nine holes of golf."

Don't make the mistake of focusing only on your patient's pain. When you see him as a person with many hopes and concerns, you'll be better able to provide complete care.

DOCUMENTATION

HOW TO DOCUMENT YOUR FINDINGS

Marie Delmonico, a 66-year-old diabetic patient, was admitted to your unit for blood glucose monitoring and regulation. Yesterday, she lost her balance and sprained her ankle—the result of chronic leg pain secondary to arthritis that she has suffered for over 5 years.

Why did the accident happen? In part, because the admitting nurse failed to document the location, duration, and extent of Mrs. Delmonico's pain. As a result, staff members were unaware of the problem and failed to take appropriate precautions.

Interviewing your patient and observing for pain are only part of pain assessment. You also have to record the data you collect on the patient's assessment form so that other members of the health-care team have the information they need to provide quality care.

In addition to helping health team members coordinate patient care, a well-designed pain assessment form:

- records baseline data
- identifies the patient's pain by location, intensity, onset, and duration
- provides a foundation for an effective care plan.

The most comprehensive and popular pain assessment form, the McGill Comprehensive Pain Questionnaire, is featured in the Appendix. Beginning at right, we'll compare other widely used assessment tools.

Note: Don't neglect to document assessment findings on other appropriate forms, such as the Kardex, your nurses' notes, and your care plan. In addition, pass on important information in report.

CHOOSING A PAIN ASSESSMENT TOOL

Used properly, a well-designed pain assessment tool provides a solid foundation for your nursing diagnoses and care plan. Any tool you select should be easy to administer, easily understood by the patient, and easily interpreted by you and other staff members. The most comprehensive tools (such as the McGill Comprehensive Pain Questionnaire) help you to:

- identify the pain source or painful area
- assess the patient's psychosocial problems
- determine factors that affect his ability to cope with pain
- plan treatment
- evaluate his response to treatment.

But depending on your patient's needs and the clinical setting, such a comprehensive tool may not be practical. The following chart features some alternatives that may better suit your needs. *Note:* If no predesigned assessment tool suits your patient's needs, consider devising your own. Incorporate the most useful elements of the tools featured here.

You and other staff members can best coordinate your efforts by consistently using the same tool. Encourage the entire staff to participate in choosing a tool, and make sure everyone knows how to use it correctly.

SIMPLE DESCRIPTIVE SCALE

Linear scale with words or numbers corresponding to the degree of pain

How to use

The patient selects the word or number along the linear scale that best represents his pain intensity.

Advantages

- Can be quickly and easily administered and interpreted
- Is easy to understand

Disadvantages

- Categorizes pain data (doesn't allow for individualized responses)
- Not reliable for comparing pain among patients, because everyone interprets pain differently

VISUAL ANALOGUE

Descriptive table with one phrase at the start (no pain) and one phrase at the end (worst pain)

How to use

The patient marks a point that best represents his pain intensity.

Advantages

- Can be quickly and easily administered and interpreted
- Is easily understood by patient
- Provides reliable results
- Allows patient to rate his pain without relating it to a specific number or word

Disadvantages

- May be too abstract for some patients

CONTINUED ON PAGE 34

Simple descriptive scales

0 1 2 3 4 5 6 7 8 9

No pain — Moderate pain — Severe pain

No pain — Mild pain — Moderate pain — Severe pain — Unbearable pain

DOCUMENTATION CONTINUED

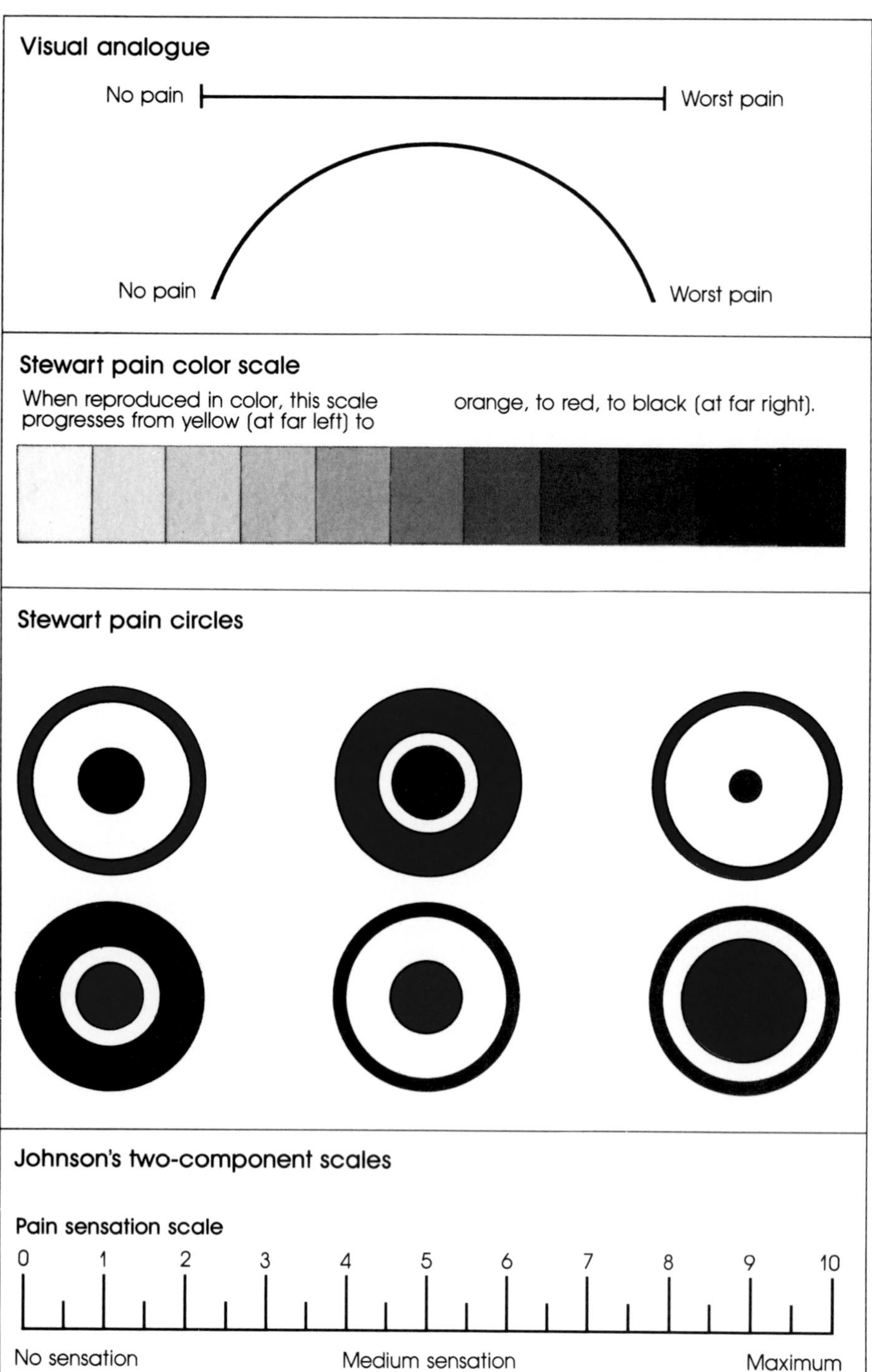

CHOOSING A PAIN ASSESSMENT TOOL
CONTINUED

STEWART PAIN COLOR SCALE

Sensory matching device consisting of colored boxes ranging from yellow (no pain) to orange, red, and black (worst possible pain)

How to use

The patient chooses the colored box that most closely corresponds to his pain.

Advantages

- May be used with a variety of patients (including children) and pain types
- Helps you evaluate the emotional component of pain
- Is quickly and easily administered

Disadvantages

- May be difficult to interpret
- Not appropriate for color-blind patients

STEWART PAIN CIRCLES

Sensory matching device consisting of six circles, three with red centers and three with black centers (see illustration at left)

How to use

The patient selects one color (black or red) to represent himself and the other to represent his pain. Then, he picks a circle that represents his pain now and his pain at its worst (if different).

Advantages

- May be used with a variety of patients (including children) and pain types
- Helps you evaluate the emotional component of pain
- Is quickly and easily administered

Disadvantages

- May be difficult to interpret
- Not appropriate for color-blind patients

ITEM CHECKLIST

Objective device that provides questions about the patient's current pain and a numerical scale to rate his responses

How to use
The patient reads the question and marks his response, according to current pain intensity.
Advantages
• Less abstract than some other tools, such as the visual analogue
• Can be easily adapted to a variety of situations by changing the questions
• Provides reliable data
• Includes physical as well as psychological factors
• Is easily administered
• Provides a numerical score for quick comparison to past ratings
Disadvantages
• Depends on the patient's ability to comprehend questions and relate them to a number scale

JOHNSON'S TWO-COMPONENT SCALES

Consists of two linear scales, one measuring pain sensation (a physical component) and the other measuring pain distress (an emotional component). As shown on page 34, the pain sensation scale rates sensation from 0 to 10. The distress scale uses words to correspond to pain intensity.
How to use
The patient circles the point on each scale that corresponds to his pain sensation and distress, respectively.
Advantages
• Defines reactions to pain and determines pain intensity
• Can be easily administered and interpreted
• Helps you evaluate the emotional component of pain
Disadvantages
• May be too ambiguous for some patients

EVALUATING YOUR ACTIONS

As part of your ongoing assessment, reevaluate your patient's pain at regular intervals, using the data provided by the pain assessment tool as a guide. For best results, encourage your patient to cooperate with the ongoing assessment by keeping a pain diary. For example, have him mark a simple descriptive scale at regular intervals.

Expect the results of your evaluation to reveal one of the following conclusions:
• The pain was properly identified, and the action plan (intervention) was effective.
• The pain was properly identified, but the intervention wasn't effective. Work with the patient to reassess and revise your care plan.
• The pain was incorrectly identified, leading to ineffective intervention. Work with the patient to revise your care plan.
• The pain was more widespread and complex than it appeared at first. As a result, your intervention was only partially effective. You need to continue your action plan for a longer time or find a new approach to pain control.

A sample flow sheet for ongoing pain assesment

PAIN FLOW SHEET

Date and time	Pain rating 0 to 10	Patient behaviors	Vital signs	Pain rating after intervention	Comments

CARE PLANS

PUTTING YOUR ASSESSMENT SKILLS TO WORK

Two years ago, Jennifer Bates, a 33-year-old sales manager with two young children, underwent bilateral mastectomies for infiltrating ductal adenocarcinoma.

Later, the pathologist reported that five axillary nodes on the left side were positive for carcinoma.

Postoperative treatment. During her 2nd week in the hospital, Mrs. Bates started chemotherapy. After discharge, she continued chemotherapy as an outpatient. A diagnostic workup following completion of therapy showed no signs of cancer.

A year later, Mrs. Bates went to her doctor complaining of fatigue and pain in her left shoulder, ribs, back, and hips. She said the pain had progressively increased over the last 6 weeks. A workup revealed bone metastasis. The doctor ordered the oral narcotic Percodan for pain.

After several weeks of outpatient chemotherapy and radiation therapy, she was admitted to the hospital. The Percodan was no longer controlling her pain.

Your assessment. Your initial pain assessment findings reveal that she:

- fears her pain won't go away.
- wants to return home.
- has throbbing pain in her shoulder, back, and legs.
- is in constant pain, despite taking a Percodan every few hours.
- uses no other pain control methods.
- finds that lying in one position exacerbates her pain.
- feels the most severe pain in the morning.
- can no longer care for her children, bathe, or drive a car.

After a thorough assessment, consult with the doctor about the medical plan for her care. Then, with Mrs. Bates' participation, formulate a nursing care plan. The chart below illustrates the plan you might devise for Mrs. Bates.

A CARE PLAN FOR MRS. BATES

Use your care plan as a basis for ongoing evaluation of the patient's condition and the effectiveness of your interventions. Update the plan regularly.

PROBLEM #1

Pain unrelieved by Percodan. Lying down makes the pain worse, as does too much walking.

Nursing diagnosis

Alteration in comfort, from breast cancer metastases to bones

Goal

To control or relieve pain

Plan of action

- Discuss analgesic regimen with doctor and other staff members: explore other pain-relief possibilities (such as radiation).
- Continue using oral analgesics as long as possible.
- Suggest and implement alternative pain-relief measures.
- Assist with frequent position changes.
- Use massage/back care every 2 to 4 hours with repositioning.
- Assess pain every 30 minutes to 1 hour after intervention.
- Plan activities with frequent rest periods.
- Create a soothing environment.

PROBLEM #2

Unable to bathe

Nursing diagnosis

Self-care deficit in bathing and hygiene

Goal

For the patient to resume bathing herself

Plan of action

- Consult with an occupational therapist for assistance with activities of daily living.
- Control pain (see problem # 1).
- Allow the patient to do as much bathing/hygiene as possible.
- Plan baths when the patient is pain-free (or as nearly pain-free as possible). For example, plan baths for 20 to 30 minutes after oral analgesic administration.

PROBLEM #3

Unable to care for children

Nursing diagnosis

Actual alterations in parenting

Goal

For the patient to resume caring for children

Plan of action

- Control pain.
- Talk with the patient and her husband about child care.
- Discuss alternatives with the patient (for example, day care).
- Contact the social service department for assistance.
- Help the patient set realistic goals for child care, based on her physical limits and the degree of pain control achieved.

PROBLEM #4

Decreased activity level secondary to pain

Nursing diagnosis

Impaired physical mobility because of metastatic bone pain

Goal

To increase the patient's mobility

Plan of action

- Consult with a physical therapist for range-of-motion activities and assistance in ambulating.
- Control pain.
- Encourage and help the patient to walk when she is pain-free (or as nearly pain-free as possible).

NONPHARMACOLOGIC THERAPIES

BASIC CONCEPTS
CONFLICTS
COGNITIVE STRATEGIES
DISTRACTION
RELAXATION
GUIDED IMAGERY
HYPNOSIS
HEAT AND COLD
MASSAGE
T.E.N.S.
BIOFEEDBACK
ACUPUNCTURE
ALTERNATIVE THERAPIES
NERVE BLOCKS
SURGERY
PAIN-CONTROL CENTERS

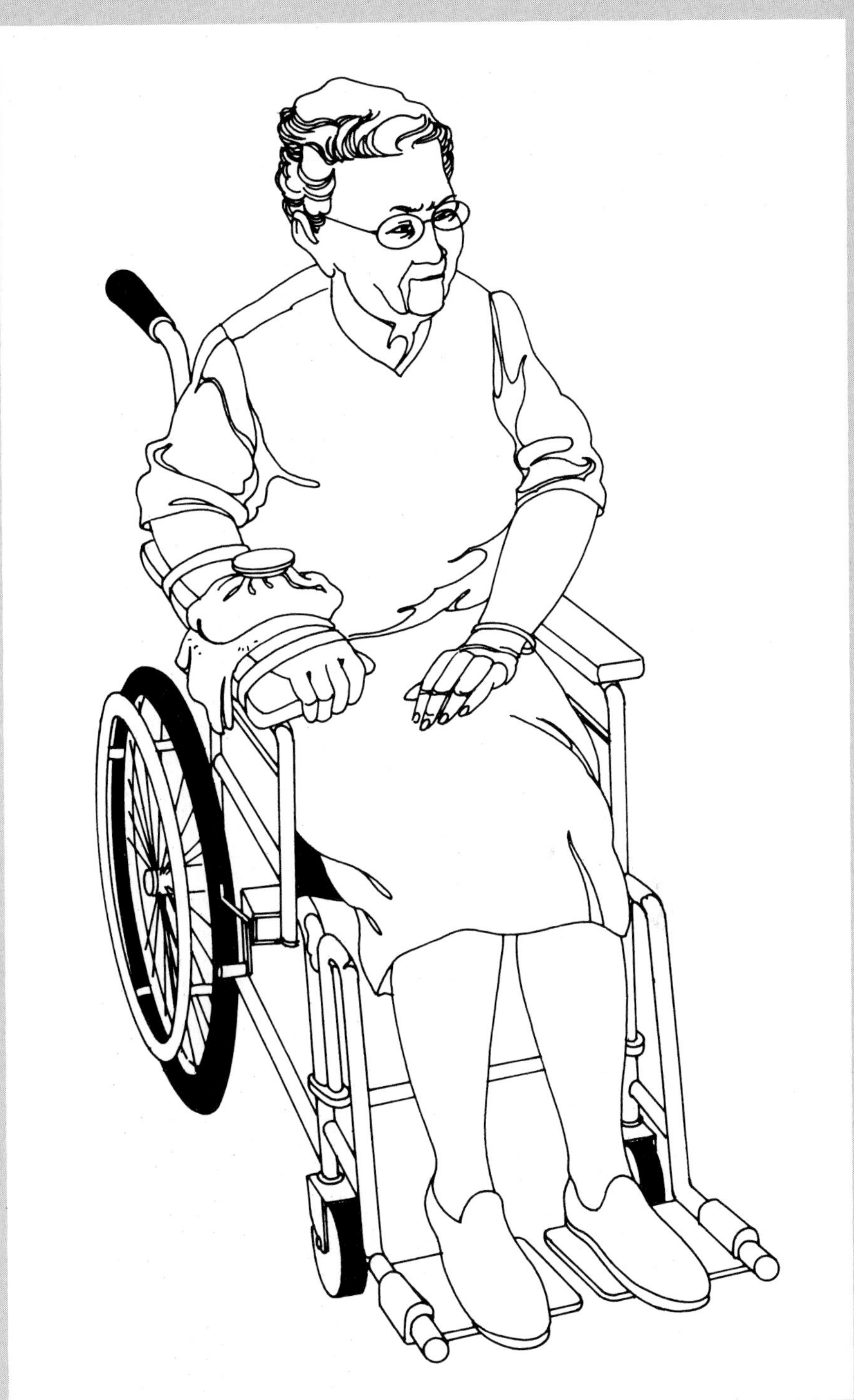

BASIC CONCEPTS

CASE IN POINT

RELIEVING PAIN WITHOUT DRUGS

Nick Wyatt, a 22-year-old law student, is an avid biker who obeys traffic laws. He keeps to the right, alerts pedestrians of his approach, wears a helmet, and, when he rides at night, wears fluorescent clothing. But sometimes doing all the right things just isn't enough. Last night, for example, Nick found himself in the wrong place at the wrong time. While biking back to his dormitory after his usual 5-mile ride, he was struck by a drunk driver who lost control of his car. The impact propelled Nick 50′ through the air. Now, he's one of your patients.

Initial care. According to his chart, Nick was unconscious when paramedics arrived at the scene. But by the time he arrived at the emergency department, he'd regained consciousness and was complaining of severe head and shoulder pain. He was also suffering from multiple abrasions on his left arm and lacerations on his face.

X-rays revealed a separated shoulder but were negative for skull fracture. A computerized axial tomography scan was also negative.

After surgery to pin his separated shoulder, Nick arrives on your unit. Because of his head injury, you observe him closely and perform frequent neurochecks.

Following doctor's orders, you give Nick acetaminophen (Tylenol), as needed. Nevertheless, he continues to complain of a severe headache. "My head feels worse, not better," he tells you. "Can't you give me anything stronger for the pain?"

You know that the doctor won't order a more potent analgesic because of Nick's head injury. But this doesn't mean you're powerless to reduce Nick's pain. You can still take steps to make him more comfortable with such simple nursing techniques as talking with him, applying ice to his head or neck, repositioning him regularly, rubbing his back, and helping him perform passive and active exercises. All these techniques can provide surprisingly effective pain relief.

Relief without drugs. Pain is modulated in the central nervous system at three levels: spine, brain stem (medulla and pons), and adrenal cortex. By intervening in ways that affect response at these levels (particularly the spinal and cortical levels), you can reduce the patient's pain.

For example, nonpharmacologic methods, such as transcutaneous electrical nerve stimulation (TENS), acupuncture, heat and cold applications, and vibration or massage, can reduce a patient's pain by stimulating the spinal cord's large nerve fibers, theoretically closing the gate to pain impulses (see pages 16 and 17). You can produce similar effects through simple comfort measures—relieving pressure by regularly turning the patient, propping him up with pillows, or giving him a back rub.

Few nonpharmacologic interventions will affect pain at the level of the medulla, which contains many opiate receptor sites. The doctor will prescribe narcotic drugs to intervene at this level.

At the cortical level, where the higher brain structures are located, behavioral modification, biofeedback, hypnosis, psychotherapy, distraction, and guided imagery can reduce a patient's pain by altering the way he perceives and responds to it emotionally. You can intervene similarly by talking to the patient about his pain, informing him about its various aspects, and offering ongoing support and reassurance.

To help a patient like Nick who can't take potent analgesic drugs, consider using one or more of these nonpharmacologic pain-relief alternatives. As we'll discuss later in this section, these alternative interventions can also effectively enhance the pain-relieving effects of analgesic drugs. Other nonpharmacologic alternatives we'll discuss include surgical procedures and pain clinics for intractable pain.

THE BENEFITS OF COLLABORATION

To decide which pain-relief measures will benefit your patient most, begin with a thorough pain assessment as detailed in the preceding section. Use your findings to help him identify some realistic pain-control goals. Then, introduce him to the pain-relief measures that will best help him reach those goals. Work closely with him as you develop a care plan, and encourage him to participate in his own care.

Collaborating with the patient can benefit him in several ways. First, it encourages him to assume responsibility for his pain, which he may be reluctant to do at first. By accepting responsibility for his care, he's likely to achieve better pain control.

Second, because the patient can choose the type of care he wishes to receive when his pain occurs, he may experience less anxiety—and, thus, less intense pain. And third, because he makes his own choices about pain relief, he's likely to be more open to trying different pain-relief measures and more willing to wait for results.

Collaborating with your patient can also help you lay the foundation for a meaningful nurse-patient relationship. This in itself lets the patient know that you believe what he tells you about his pain and want to help him. Furthermore, studies show that talking with a pain sufferer, regardless of the topic, will make him feel better. According to some reports, talking to the patient about his difficulties for 15 minutes can relieve his pain for at least an hour. What's more, by taking time to elicit the patient's ideas and values about his pain, and planning pain-relief interventions accordingly, you let him know that you accept and respect the way he responds to pain. As a result, he expends less energy trying to control his pain behavior in order to meet what he perceives as your expectations. Because he's more relaxed and less defensive about his behavior, he experiences less pain.

IMPLEMENTING A PAIN-RELIEF PROGRAM

Because pain is so highly subjective, you must plan treatment that meets your patient's particular needs. These guidelines will help you plan an individualized program.

• *Use pain-relief measures preventively.* Relieving severe pain isn't easy. And the longer a patient suffers from pain, the less likely he'll be to respond to your interventions. So try to start pain-relief measures before the pain begins, or as soon as possible after its onset. For example, administer an analgesic or suggest that the patient start a distraction technique prior to a dressing change or other painful procedure. Or suggest a relaxation technique or guided imagery as soon as his pain begins or worsens. For predictable, recurring pain, administer analgesics at regularly scheduled times.

Such preventive approaches will protect your patient from what researchers call the *pain disaster threshold.* According to research findings, the patient who experiences severe and long-lasting pain will eventually lose control of his emotions and behavior. The pain disaster threshold varies among patients. But once a patient reaches it, he may never again regain control over his pain and even minor pain may become unbearable.

• *Use two or more pain-relief methods simultaneously.* Because a single pain-relief measure rarely controls pain effectively, help your patient choose several methods that will complement and enhance one another. Examples of some effective combinations are analgesic drugs and relaxation, application of ice and distraction, and cutaneous stimulation and guided imagery.

• *Respect the patient's ideas about pain relief.* Some patients rely on unscientific practices. Others seek help from individuals outside medicine. For example, you've probably cared for an arthritic patient who believes that a copper bracelet gives him relief, or for a patient who turns to faith healing for pain control. As long as these nontraditional practices don't harm your patient, respect his decision to use them. *Important:* Never doubt the reality of a patient's pain just because he gets relief from nontraditional therapies.

• *Build upon the patient's strengths.* You may be able to build on techniques the patient has used in the past to effectively relieve his pain. For example, if he's used relaxation or distraction techniques, help him perfect them and suggest additional ones.

• *Choose pain-relief measures appropriate to his ability to participate.* Some patients, because of mental or physical problems, can't participate actively in pain-control measures. Others, because of depression, lack motivation. For these patients, analgesic drug therapy is one approach that requires little, if any, participation. But you can also modify other techniques. For example, instead of having the

CONTINUED ON PAGE 40

BASIC CONCEPTS CONTINUED

IMPLEMENTING A PAIN-RELIEF PROGRAM CONTINUED

patient perform cutaneous stimulation, do it for him. Or use such passive distraction techniques as having the patient listen to music through earphones.

• *Let the patient evaluate his pain.* Only he knows what kind of pain (and how much) he's experiencing. So believe him when he says his pain is severe, and start pain-relief measures. Also, ask him to periodically evaluate his pain program. Make him the authority on its effectiveness.

• *Modify the pain program, as needed, but do it gradually.* A patient may eventually rely so heavily on a specific pain-relief measure that he'd feel insecure without it. However, some measures, no matter how effective, must be withdrawn if they cause complications. Long-term use of some parenteral narcotics, for example, can damage muscle tissue. If you must change the patient's pain program for such a reason, do so gradually. Allow him to continue using the old measure while he evaluates the effectiveness of the new one.

• *Keep trying.* Tell the patient from the start that the new program may not work immediately. If after several tries the program proves ineffective, reassure him that you'll try to find an alternative. Start by reviewing your assessment findings for pain factors or influences you may have overlooked; implement new methods you may have omitted; modify previously unsuccessful techniques; and discuss new approaches with the patient. If all your efforts fail, consider referring the patient to a pain clinic or a holistic health center. If his pain is associated with a terminal illness, consider referring him to a hospice program.

THE LITTLE THINGS THAT COUNT

You know about pain's vicious cycle: pain elicits fear and anxiety in a patient, which in turn worsens and possibly prolongs his pain. Analgesics can stop the cycle, of course. But don't forget about the little things that count. For example, a friendly, understanding chat with your patient, plus some basic nursing interventions, can significantly reduce his pain. So the next time you care for a patient in pain, try to enhance his prescribed medical regimen with some of these techniques:

COMFORT MEASURES

• *Reposition the patient* periodically—turn him from side to side or move him from a reclining to a sitting position—to reduce muscle spasm and tension and to relieve pressure on bony prominences. Such movement also helps prevent painful joint stiffness.

• *Maintain proper body alignment* to prevent painful contractures.

• *Assure adequate bed rest or immobilize a painful part,* if appropriate, to enhance healing and reduce pain.

• *Elevate an extremity,* if appropriate, to reduce swelling, inflammation, and pain. For example, place pillows under a patient's casted arm.

• *Perform back massage* to help relax tense muscles throughout his body.

ENVIRONMENTAL CONSIDERATIONS

• *Eliminate as many noxious stimuli as possible* from the patient's room (for example, bright lights, bright colors, and loud noises).

• *Provide the patient with quiet, soothing surroundings.* For example, dim the lights; draw the blinds; and make sure the call light, telephone, water pitcher, and other necessary items are within his reach. Discourage visits from individuals who may upset him.

PATIENT TEACHING

• *Reduce the patient's fear of the unknown* by doing preoperative teaching to reduce his anxiety and lessen his postoperative pain. Also, tell the patient what kind of pain he can anticipate, when it's likely to occur, and how long it may last.

• *Inform him about his options for pain relief.* And tell him how he can use each method most effectively. Encourage him to take control of his pain experience.

EMOTIONAL SUPPORT

• *Spend time with your patient.* Pain sufferers often feel lonely, depressed, and afraid. Even if you have only a few minutes to spare, *sit* with him (don't stand in the doorway or at the foot of his bed) and ask him how he's feeling. Lean toward him, and listen attentively to his responses. Make sure your body language communicates your concern and interest.

• *Use direct eye contact* whenever you talk with him.

• *Help his family and friends understand his emotional needs.* Include them in your teaching. Keeping them informed of the patient's status reduces their anxiety, too.

CONFLICTS

WHEN PROFESSIONALS DISAGREE

Alison Kendell, age 44, is a housewife and mother of two who was admitted to the hospital after experiencing abdominal pain for several weeks. When her diagnostic workup showed a severely inflamed gallbladder, she underwent a cholecystectomy. Though the surgery went smoothly, Mrs. Kendell developed postoperative atelectasis and wound infection.

The doctor ordered the following postoperative care: ambulation three times a day and incentive spirometry four times a day or as needed to treat the atelectasis. For the wound, he ordered dressing changes three times a day and the following pain medication as needed: for severe pain, 75 to 100 mg of Demerol I.M. every 3 to 4 hours; for moderate pain, 50 mg of Demerol I.M. every 3 to 4 hours; for mild pain, after the patient can tolerate fluids, 650 mg of Tylenol P.O. every 3 to 4 hours.

Initial pain control. When you check on Mrs. Kendell at the start of your shift, she complains of pain that she says worsens during dressing changes and when she walks. To relieve it, you give her the maximum dose of Demerol (100 mg) at the most frequent intervals (every 3 hours) ordered by the doctor. At the end of your 12-hour shift, you've given Mrs. Kendell a total of 400 mg of Demerol I.M. As evidenced by her physical activity—three walks to and from the sun-room and frequent spirometer use—these doses have effectively controlled her pain.

A different approach. The nurse on the night shift, however, responds to Mrs. Kendell's complaints differently. She gives Mrs. Kendell the *minimum* dose of Demerol (50 mg) at the *least frequent* intervals ordered (every 4 hours). Between doses, she gives the patient Tylenol, as ordered. At the end of this nurse's shift, Mrs. Kendell has received only 150 mg of Demerol.

By the time you arrive on the unit the next morning, Mrs. Kendell is tense and anxious. Her pain, she says, is so severe that she can't breathe deeply. She's reluctant to walk even the short distance to the bathroom. "I was doing so well yesterday. What happened?" she asks. "Is my infection getting worse?"

A quick look at the night nurse's notes tells you why Mrs. Kendell has so much physical discomfort and emotional distress. Understanding why the night nurse's care differed so dramatically from yours may not be so easy. Yet such conflicts in the assessment and management of pain are far from uncommon among nurses and other health-care professionals.

Reasons for conflict. Why the lack of uniform standards in pain management? Many factors play a part. No matter how objective you try to be, your personal opinion of the patient—and her attitude toward you and nursing in general—affects how you interpret and respond to her pain. Other explanations for diverging approaches include:

- differences in education, training, and experience concerning pain and pain control
- differing opinions about how and when patients should achieve treatment goals
- confusion about the role of nurses in pain management
- differing opinions about alternative pain therapies
- differing beliefs (or misconceptions) about the nature of pain and about such drug-related issues as addiction, tolerance, and dependence
- poor communication.

Regardless of the reasons, these conflicts stand in the way of effective pain management. When the staff works at cross-purposes, the patient receives inconsistent care that may shake her confidence in you and prolong or intensify her suffering. All your patients are entitled to well-coordinated, quality care. To discover how you can ensure it, read the following pages.

Doctor's orders: Open to interpretation

If the doctor wrote these orders for your patient, how would you decide which drug—and what dosage—she needs?

MEMORIAL HOSPITAL
Lansdale, Pa.

10/1	Postop orders (con't)	Alison Kendell #10568 Room 335A
	Demerol 75-100 mg I.M. q 3-4 hours	
	p.r.n. severe pain	
	Demerol 50 mg I.M. q 3-4 hours	
	p.r.n. moderate pain	
	Tylenol 650 mg P.O. q 3-4 hours	
	p.r.n. mild pain	
	M. Goldman M.D.	

CONFLICTS CONTINUED

ASSURING CONSISTENT CARE

Identifying and working through the reasons for a nursing staff's conflicts over managing a patient's pain is the first step toward a workable solution. For best results, hold a care conference with other members of the health-care team—nursing as well as nonnursing personnel. Work at resolving the current conflict. Then try to arrive at ways to avoid future conflicts and to ensure a consistent, systematic approach to each patient's pain care.

Start by identifying a pain-relief goal that everyone agrees on. For Mrs. Kendell, that goal might be to walk four times a day with a minimal increase in pain during the activity.

Then, give staff members a chance to express their beliefs and attitudes about the patient's pain as well as pain in general. Make sure they realize that they're entitled to their beliefs and won't be criticized or judged for expressing them. The staff's responses may provide an opportunity for some continuing education about myths and misconceptions surrounding pain. For example, in Mrs. Kendell's case, the night nurse may have felt that she was protecting the patient from drug addiction by giving her the minimum Demerol dosage ordered. Explain that drug addiction rarely occurs under such circumstances. (We'll discuss this issue in detail in Section 4.) If your hospital has a pain-control nurse clinician, ask her to sit in on the conference. Arrange for some inservice education classes on pain, too.

Assessing the problem. Review the patient's chart to determine his current physical status and response to treatment. Then, ask each staff member to identify what she sees as appropriate pain-management goals. Also, identify the patient's views and expectations about his pain and what he perceives as appropriate goals for its management. Mrs. Kendell, for example, expected only minimal postoperative pain and was unprepared for such possible complications as atelectasis and wound infection.

Analyze the staff's approaches to pain relief and the patient's response to each. Select the approaches that produce the most desirable and beneficial patient response. (For Mrs. Kendell, the maximum dosage of Demerol best supported her pain-relief goals.) Then, try to develop a compromise care plan that's agreed to by the patient and staff members and that provides the patient with optimum pain control.

A compromise care plan. For Mrs. Kendell, you might agree to give 100 mg of Demerol about 30 minutes before each dressing change and ambulation. At bedtime and during the night, you'd give her 50 to 75 mg. Then you'd assess her response and adjust the dosage accordingly. In addition, you might ask the doctor to substitute a stronger oral medication, such as Percodan or Tylox*, for the Tylenol.

To further encourage consistent care, ask the doctor to clarify his orders. For example, ask how he defines *mild* and *moderate* pain and how he expects you to assess the difference.

Once you have a care plan, develop a way for all staff members to assess, diagnose, and treat the patient's pain. For details, see the information at right.

Despite all your efforts, some staff members may remain adamant about their beliefs on pain and care approaches. If these staff members fail to compromise, tactfully ask if they want to be assigned to another patient whose care needs are more compatible with their personal beliefs.

Staff conferences: A chance to resolve conflicts

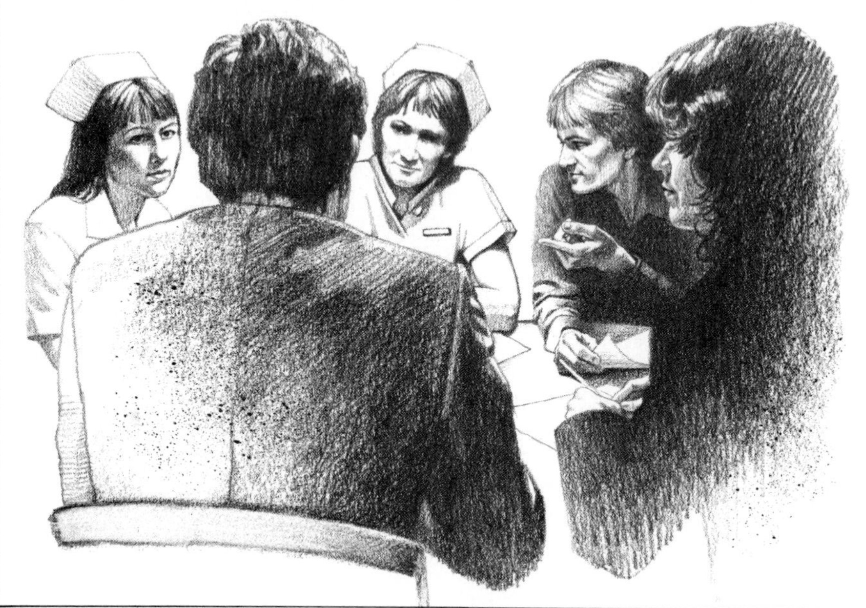

*Not available in Canada

COGNITIVE STRATEGIES

OBJECTIVE PAIN ASSESSMENT

To provide your patient with consistent and effective pain care, you and other staff members must assess his pain objectively, using consistent standards of reference. Follow these suggestions for developing a standardized pain-assessment tool.

- Work with other nurses on your unit to establish standard pain-assessment criteria. Suggest a pain-rating scale of 0 to 10, for example, with 0 representing no pain and 10 the worst pain. Whenever you ask a patient about his pain, record the pain-rating number that he specifies.
- Correlate pain-medication doses to the patient's pain rating. For example, if Mrs. Kendell rated her pain at 8 to 10, you'd give her 100 mg of pain medication; for a pain rating of 6 to 8, 75 mg; 4 to 6, 50 mg. Assess the patient's response and adjust the dose, if necessary.
- Use the assessment tool systematically and record information on the patient's chart and medication Kardex.

Once you've chosen an assessment tool, get the most from it by doing the following:

- Assess your patient's pain *before* you intervene with a pain-relief method. Then, reassess his pain afterward, to evaluate the treatment's effectiveness.
- When necessary, alter your approach: for example, try a new pain-relief method or alter the patient's dosage schedule (with the doctor's approval). Consult your patient, however, before you make any changes. He's more likely to agree to your suggestions if he's part of the decision-making process.
- Report the effectiveness of pain-relief methods at the change-of-shift report.

HELPING YOUR PATIENT HELP HIMSELF

Many patients—and even some nurses—believe that drug therapy is the only effective way to relieve pain. Not true. Most of us have the innate ability to harness our mental powers to block pain at the cortical level. By using such techniques as distraction, relaxation, guided imagery, and hypnosis, a patient can exert some control over pain perception. Because these techniques employ his ability to think and imagine, we'll call them *cognitive strategies.*

Of these strategies, distraction and relaxation are the simplest to teach and use. Hypnosis and guided imagery, which are closely related, require more specialized training and practice to be effective.

What do cognitive strategies have in common? First of all, they're virtually risk-free. Second, they let the patient participate actively in his pain relief, giving him a sense of control over his condition. Once mastered, most strategies can be used as needed, without any special equipment or assistance.

As you read about these strategies on the following pages, you'll probably discover that you're already incorporating many of them into your daily nursing care. For example, whenever you strike up a conversation with a patient during a venipuncture, you're using distraction to shift his attention from the painful site. Similarly, if you encourage your patient to perform a breathing exercise during a painful debridement, you're using relaxation to ease his pain.

When you introduce these pain-relief techniques to your patient, you may be surprised to learn that he, too, is familiar with them. Many patients instinctively develop pain-relief methods that mimic or incorporate one or more cognitive strategies. For example, a patient may cope with pain by counting the number of bricks in a wall, flowers on a drape, or letters in a word. Another patient may recite an oath or poem or repeat a word or phrase. Still another patient may turn to a hobby, such as sculpture or wood carving.

Never underestimate your patient's ability to minimize his pain. Instead, use it to individualize his pain-relief program.

TEACHING TIPS

On the following pages, you'll find out more about such cognitive strategies as distraction, relaxation, and guided imagery, which you can teach your patient for pain relief. As you employ these methods, ensure good results by observing the following points.

The first stop: An open mind. Before you can teach your patient to use a cognitive strategy, you must convince him that it can help him. If he's already practicing distraction, imagery, or relaxation to some degree, he'll probably welcome your efforts and eagerly try new techniques. But if he's unfamiliar with them, he may resist your efforts for these reasons:

- He believes that only medication relieves pain.
- He believes that his pain is too severe to respond to such strategies.
- He suspects that you don't believe he has pain or that you think his pain is less severe than it is.

Gain your patient's confidence by reassuring him that you know

CONTINUED ON PAGE 44

COGNITIVE STRATEGIES CONTINUED

TEACHING TIPS CONTINUED

he has pain and want to help him. Then, discuss his options with him and help him choose a technique that he feels comfortable with. If appropriate, explain that these techniques will accompany other pain-relief measures, such as drug therapy. And support and encourage him throughout the learning process.

Choosing the right time. If possible, begin instructing your patient when his pain is absent or mild. Plan his nursing care so that he has plenty of time to practice the technique before his pain occurs. Practicing will increase his skill and improve his confidence.

Some patients feel less self-conscious about practicing these techniques if you practice along with them; others prefer to practice in private. Be sure to ask your patient which method he prefers.

Instruct the patient to begin the technique before a painful procedure or as soon as his pain begins. For example, a postoperative patient may begin to use guided imagery or distraction before you perform a painful dressing change.

Special Note:

Don't hesitate to teach a patient a noninvasive technique such as distraction *during* an acute pain episode. Although pain will decrease his ability to learn, it can also increase his motivation.

Make sure you inform the patient's family about the techniques he's learning, so they can encourage and support him. Also, document your teaching in your nurses' notes and patient care plan so other staff members can reinforce your efforts.

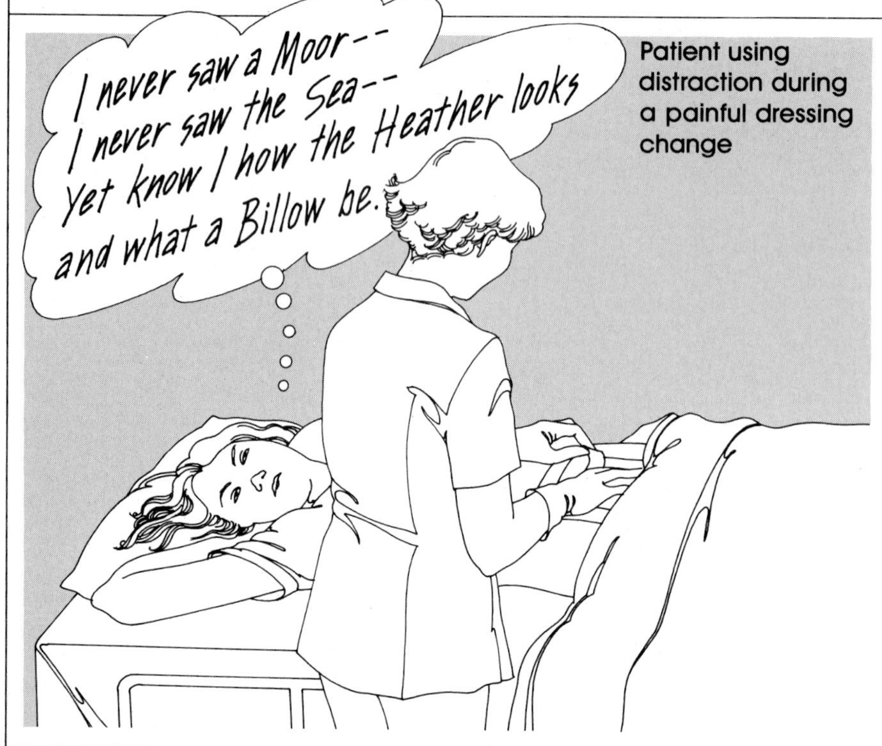

Patient using distraction during a painful dressing change

DISTRACTION

A SIMPLE BUT EFFECTIVE TECHNIQUE

Distraction is probably the easiest noninvasive pain-relief technique to teach your patient because it's one that you use every day without even thinking about it. Although most effective for relieving acute pain, distraction can also be effective against chronic pain.

With distraction, your patient learns to focus his attention on something other than his pain. Reading a book, watching a televised sports event, or simply engaging in conversation are some of the most common examples of distraction. As the patient concentrates on one of these activities, it becomes the center of his awareness. Although the exact mechanism is unclear, the result is that the patient feels less pain.

Distraction relieves pain only while the patient practices the technique. Afterward, pain returns undiminished.

Unfortunately, the effectiveness of this simple technique can lead to misconceptions about the patient's pain. When distraction successfully relieves pain, the patient's doctor or family may doubt its severity. Or a nurse may be confused over a patient's request for pain medication if, moments before, he had been talking happily and effortlessly with his wife or daughter. If the nurse refuses to give him medication based on her observations, the patient may suffer needlessly.

You can avoid such unfortunate misunderstandings by familiarizing yourself with distraction and educating other staff members about it. The information that follows will help.

TEACHING DISTRACTION TECHNIQUES

Use one or more of these techniques to distract your patient from his pain.

Music therapy. If your patient likes music, ask his family to provide a tape recorder with a headset and cassettes of his favorite music. Tell him to sit or lie down in a comfortable position, with his legs and arms uncrossed and relaxed, while he listens to the music through the headset.

Depending on his preference, he can either close his eyes and concentrate on the music or stare at a nearby object. To combine music therapy with imagery (see pages 48 and 49), suggest that he imagine himself floating or drifting with the music. Or have him focus on images suggested by the music or on a pleasant scene of his own choosing.

Because rhythmic movement can also serve as distraction, tell the patient to keep time with the music by tapping a finger or foot, slapping his thigh, or nodding his head.

Advise the patient to keep his finger on the recorder's volume control dial. If his pain increases, encourage him to increase the volume; when the pain subsides, instruct him to decrease it.

This distraction technique has several advantages:

- It provides a demanding auditory stimulus for the patient without disturbing others.
- A tired, sedated, or passive patient can use it effectively.
- The patient can respond to varying pain intensities by adjusting the volume.

Singing. This technique also makes use of rhythm as a distractor. Have the patient select a song he likes. Then, tell him to:

- mouth the words, exaggerating the lip movement, while he sings it in his mind. (Children and some adults may want to sing out loud.)
- concentrate all his attention on the words and rhythm of the song. (Closing his eyes may help.)
- sing faster or louder when the pain intensifies; slower when the pain subsides.

Note: Sing with him, if you wish.

Special Note:

If your patient doesn't like music, substitute recordings of comedy routines, stories, or sports events.

Rhythmic breathing. This technique may appeal to a patient who prefers a more structured distraction technique. Tell your patient to:

- stare at you or an object and inhale slowly and deeply.
- exhale slowly.
- continue breathing slowly and comfortably (but not too deeply) while you count: "In, 2, 3—out, 2, 3, 4." Have him count silently as you count aloud.
- concentrate on the *feel* of his breathing. He might want to close his eyes and imagine the air moving slowly in and out of his lungs.
- count silently to himself after establishing a comfortable, rhythmic pattern.

If he begins to feel breathless, tell him to breathe more slowly or take a deep breath.

If rhythmic breathing alone isn't sufficient distraction to relieve his pain, make the technique more complex. Suggest that he massage the painful area (or the contralateral area) with a stroking or circular motion as he breathes. Or tell him to raise his arm as he inhales and lower it as he exhales. Also suggest that he inhale through his nose and exhale through his mouth.

Description. Give your patient a photo, and ask him to describe every detail or to make up a story about it. To avoid influencing his comments, close your eyes or look away from the photo. Then, ask him questions based on his description.

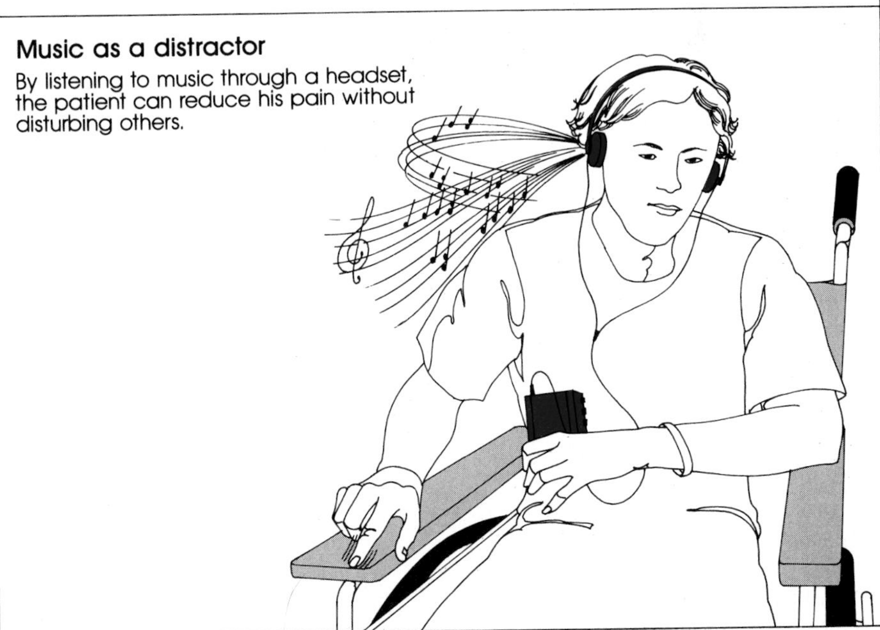

Music as a distractor

By listening to music through a headset, the patient can reduce his pain without disturbing others.

DISTRACTION CONTINUED

DISTRACTION GUIDELINES

Unlike most other cognitive strategies, distraction diminishes a patient's pain regardless of whether he believes in its effectiveness. But to best help a skeptical patient, point out instances when distraction helped him and encourage him to consciously use the distraction technique whenever his pain occurs. Follow these guidelines to help him develop an individualized strategy for pain relief.

• *Explain benefits and limitations.* Tell him that distraction is a simple but effective technique that he can use at will, whenever pain returns or intensifies. But also advise him that the pain will probably return when he stops the distraction exercise. Inform him that distraction can be tiring. The resulting fatigue may intensify his pain after the exercise.

Make sure he understands that distraction is a *short-term* pain-relief measure—most patients can't use it for long periods without becoming bored or tired. An exercise such as rhythmic breathing, for example, can be especially tiring. Reassure him that other pain-relief measures, such as medication, are available for use along with distraction.

• *Help him choose a distraction stimulus (distractor).* Ask him about his interests or hobbies. He'll be distracted most effectively by something that interests him. If he's used distraction before or if he's developed his own distraction technique for his current pain, build upon that.

If your patient is in acute pain and assessment of his special interests isn't practical, let him choose from among several different distraction techniques, such as breathing rhythmically, describing pictures, or singing a song.

• *If possible, use distractors that involve more than one of the patient's senses.* The most effective distractors are those that engage the patient's senses of hearing, sight, or touch.

• *Encourage him to use distractors that require more concentration when his pain intensifies.* A simple distraction like listening to music may help the patient cope with mild pain. But if his pain worsens, a more complex distractor (such as a chess game) that requires his complete attention may be more effective.

• *If possible, make rhythm and repetition part of the distraction technique.* Many patients have great success with rhythmic breathing patterns: taking shallow or deep breaths; breathing from the chest or abdomen; breathing slowly and deeply; or controlling the length of time for inhalation or exhalation. However, when rhythmic breathing is impractical (as for obese patients and those with pulmonary disorders), incorporate background music, finger tapping, or a repeated word or phrase into the patient's distraction strategy.

• *Avoid pain-related distractors.* Distraction may be ineffective if the patient looks at his painful body part, watches a painful procedure, or even envisions such scenes. If he's using a distraction technique while undergoing a painful procedure, advise him to stare at a spot on the wall.

Special Note:

During periods of intense pain, the patient's ability to concentrate diminishes. To avoid frustrating him, choose a distractor that's simple enough for him to concentrate on under the circumstances.

RELAXATION

STRESS, PAIN, AND RELAXATION

Relaxation is one of the most widely used cognitive strategies for acute as well as chronic pain. One reason for its popularity is that it effectively alters autonomic nervous system (ANS) activity, thus affecting the patient's physiologic response to stress.

Normally, when a stressful condition such as pain occurs, ANS activity causes muscle tension and an increase in heart rate, blood pressure, and respiratory rate. All of these responses intensify pain.

Relaxation can diminish a patient's pain by minimizing ANS activity. It may also reduce muscle tension and contractions that can cause pain. Among other desirable effects, it may enhance comfort measures and other pain-relief interventions and reduce the patient's anxiety.

Some precautions. Though relaxation is noninvasive and virtually risk-free, you may need to consult the doctor before using it with some patients. A cardiac patient, for example, may respond so well to relaxation that the doctor will need to adjust his medication schedule.

Get the doctor's permission before using relaxation with a severely depressed or psychotic patient. Then, proceed with caution. Such a patient may need to feel in control of himself. Relaxation may give him a sense of losing control, causing anxiety.

If you perform relaxation with a respiratory patient, minimize or eliminate deep breathing exercises, such as those used in progressive muscle relaxation, which we'll discuss on the following page. These exercises could exacerbate his preexisting condition.

Finally, if your patient wears contact lenses, ask him to remove them before he begins a relaxation exercise. Explain that because he'll keep his eyes closed during the exercise, his contact lenses won't be lubricated adequately. As a result, he'd risk corneal abrasion, or the lenses could adhere to his corneas.

Other considerations. Relaxation is especially useful when a patient is waiting for his pain medication to work and when he faces a painful procedure. However, before teaching your patient relaxation, inform him that immediate results are unlikely (unless he's been using relaxation regularly).

Because relaxation is a learned behavior, your patient must practice it regularly—daily, if possible—for best results.

Plan your nursing care so he has time each day to practice relaxation. During that time, ensure his privacy. Close his door, or hang a sign on it to prevent interruptions. If possible, take him to a more private area, such as the chapel or a conference room. For more guidelines, read what follows.

THE RELAXATION RESPONSE: FIRST STEPS

Relaxation techniques include such meditative methods as transcendental meditation (TM), yoga, and Zen Buddhism; such autogenic therapies as biofeedback; and self-hypnosis. Though each technique is unique, certain elements are common to each. All of them aim for the same effect: the *relaxation response,* a state of deep relaxation accompanied by decreased blood pressure, heart rate, respiratory rate, and muscle tension. While relaxed, the patient may feel general or localized warmth, heaviness, lightness, or tingling.

The following are essential prerequisites for each technique:

• *a quiet environment.*

• *a mental device.* Have the patient choose a sound, word, or phrase that he can repeat silently or out loud. Or tell him to stare at an object in the room.

• *a passive attitude.* Encourage him to allow relaxation to occur naturally. Explain that distracting thoughts are likely to occur, especially during the learning stages; they don't mean that he's performing the technique incorrectly. If distracting thoughts occur, he should try to disregard them and continue concentrating.

• *a comfortable position.* Make sure his muscles are as relaxed as possible. Sitting upright or with his legs crossed in the lotus position are positions that reduce muscular tension. Or if he wants to induce sleep, he may lie down.

TEACHING PROGRESSIVE MUSCLE RELAXATION

The most commonly used relaxation exercise is progressive muscle relaxation (PMR), which your patient performs by systematically tensing and relaxing muscle groups. Teach him PMR by following these guidelines, or use a commercially prepared tape.

• Tell him to focus on a muscle group, such as the muscles in his hands. Have him tense his forearm muscles and make a fist. When his muscles are tense, tell him to note the sensation.

• After 5 to 7 seconds, signal him to release his fist and relax his muscles. Urge him to concentrate on the difference between the relaxed and tensed states.

• Then tell him to concentrate on another group of muscles. Continue the procedure until he's tensed and relaxed the major muscle groups throughout his body. *Note:* For best results, choose a systematic approach. Incorporate deep breathing with chest relaxation.

Completing the exercise. The simplest way to end the exercise includes these three steps: Tell him to slowly open his eyes; then to stretch, as if awakening from a deep sleep; and finally, to walk around until he feels alert.

Alternatives. For pain that occurs suddenly, your patient should know some shorter relaxation exercises that produce quick results. For example, a patient who's undergoing a lumbar puncture might benefit from one of these 10-second exercises:

• Tell him to relax his lower jaw as if he were starting to yawn and to rest his tongue on the bottom of his mouth. Then, suggest that he breathe slowly and rhythmically through his mouth: inhaling, exhaling, then resting. Advise him not to even think of words.

• Or instruct him to close his eyes and imagine a small star about 1" from the tip of his nose. Then, tell him to breathe deeply and slowly four times through his mouth while focusing on the star.

GUIDED IMAGERY

USING IMAGERY TO CONTROL PAIN

Similar to hypnosis, guided imagery is a cognitive strategy that allows the patient to use his imagination to create images that decrease pain intensity by focusing his attention elsewhere. Unlike hypnosis, however, guided imagery is a technique that most patients can learn quickly and perform easily, either on their own or with assistance. By following the guidelines on these two pages, you can help your patient learn this effective pain-control strategy.

In part, imagery is effective because it can produce physiologic changes. For example, think how you've reacted to watching a frightening movie scene. Most likely, you experienced such sympathetic nervous system responses as rapid respirations and heart rate. Under special circumstances, simply recalling the scene could cause the same responses long after you viewed the movie. Similarly, imagining how a lemon tastes can make your mouth water.

For pain relief, imagery makes use of the mind's ability to affect physiologic response as well as pain perception. And, like other cognitive strategies, imagery promotes muscle relaxation and decreases anxiety. For best results, your patient should practice imagery techniques regularly. Read what follows for details on making imagery work for him.

TAKING THE FIRST STEPS

To use guided imagery most effectively, the patient must be able and willing to create images in his mind. In addition, he must create images that are appropriate for relieving his pain. Here's how to acquaint your patient with the technique.

Patient teaching. If your patient is hesitant about using guided imagery, explain that the technique is just an extension of everyday thoughts. Point out that when he talks with a stranger on the telephone, he probably imagines what that person looks like. Similarly, when he closes his eyes, he can probably envision every detail of his kitchen or living room. You might also ask him to recall the last time he gave someone directions and how he imagined every landmark as he described it. When he realizes that he routinely uses imagery without a second thought, he'll probably feel more comfortable with the technique.

To help your patient learn guided imagery techniques, tape-record a session you conduct with him or give him a commercial recording. This way, he can practice imagery without assistance.

While you talk to your patient, determine if he has any fears or misconceptions that make him reluctant to try guided imagery. For example, he may be afraid that imagery will draw him into a trancelike state from which he'll never awaken. To dispel this misconception, tell him that before each session he can determine how long he'd like the guided imagery to last. For most patients, 15 to 20 minutes is long enough; however, the interval may also be affected by the length of time necessary for a painful procedure. Reassure him that he can stop performing imagery at will.

Image selection. If your patient agrees to try imagery, help him choose an appropriate image; however, make sure that it's relaxing and pleasant for him. Keep in mind that everyone has different ideas about what's pleasant. A country scene, for example, may provoke anxiety in someone with asthma or hay fever. Similarly, someone who sunburns easily may find a beach scene unpleasant.

For best results, encourage the patient to choose images based on his experiences, since such images will be most meaningful and vivid for him. He can select a particular experience or choose aspects of several experiences and develop a composite image.

To increase the image's vividness, advise him to engage most or all of his senses. For instance, if he chooses a mountain scene, tell him to imagine feeling a cool breeze, hearing the wind rustling the leaves, tasting fresh spring water, and seeing brightly colored autumn foliage. Most important, encourage him to imagine how relaxed and peaceful he'd feel in such surroundings.

HOW TO PERFORM GUIDED IMAGERY

Once you've decided on an appropriate sensory image, prepare your patient to begin the exercise. Encourage him to find a comfortable position, take a deep breath, and try to relax. Eliminate interruptions and create a soothing environment by dimming the lights, drawing the blinds, and minimizing noise. (Or if your patient has chosen a sunny scene, you might enhance the image by opening the blinds.) Then, follow the guidelines below to perform a guided imagery exercise.

Note: Using a relaxation exercise may help prepare your patient to begin guided imagery.

- Begin by telling your patient to close his eyes and concentrate intensely on the predetermined image. Then tell him to describe all the possible sensations suggested by the image.
- If he's hesitant about describing sensations, ask specific questions; for example, if he chose a mountain scene, ask: "What do you see from the cabin? What color is the sky? Is the ground firm or soft? Can you hear animals or running water?"
- If he's still having trouble responding, introduce the image gradually by slowly constructing the scene. For example, ask him what items he packed for his mountain vacation, how long the drive was, what the cabin looked like when he arrived, and how he felt at the time. This helps the patient relax and draws him gradually into the image.
- After the predetermined time, instruct your patient to arouse himself from his deeply relaxed and pain-free state. You can end the session in several ways, but the most common method is to have the patient count silently from one to three. Tell him to take a deep breath on the last count, open his eyes, and say, "I feel alert and relaxed."

Note: Some patients feel drowsy after using guided imagery.

Special Note:

As you work through the exercise, be careful not to interpret the patient's sensations for him or to interject information that may be inappropriate or disturbing to him. Instead, make suggestions and ask open-ended questions that will spur his imagination.

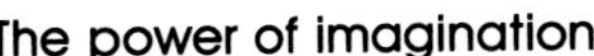

The power of imagination

By imagining every detail of a mountain scene—sights, sounds, smells, and other sensations—and evoking positive emotions, the patient minimizes pain sensations.

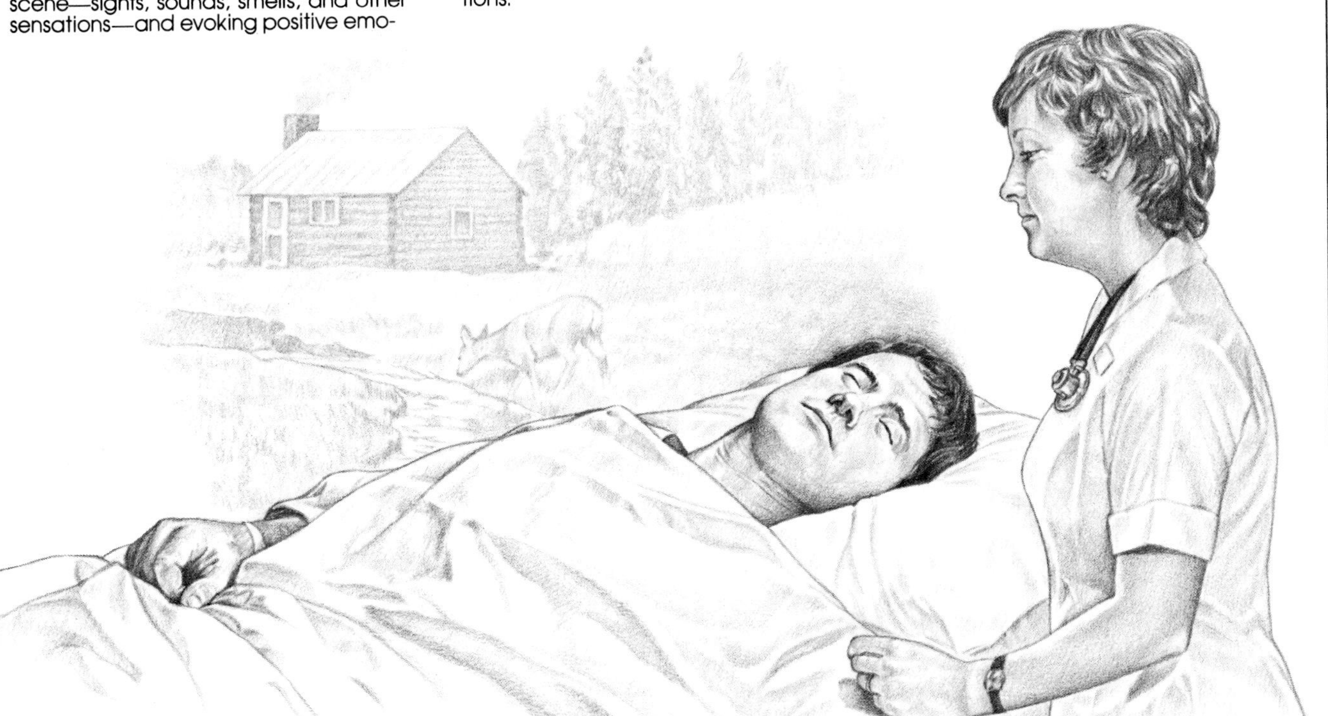

HYPNOSIS

USING HYPNOSIS TO CONTROL PAIN

Hypnosis has come a long way since Anton Mesmer practiced his so-called animal magnetism on wealthy 18th-century Europeans. Today, health-care workers are beginning to recognize the medical value of hypnosis, particularly to control chronic pain.

Hypnosis is an altered state of consciousness in which concentration is focused and distraction minimized. Under hypnosis, a person is highly suggestible, receptive to possibilities presented by a trained hypnotherapist.

Although scientists have been studying hypnosis for some time, no one really knows how it relieves pain. Apparently, hypnosis doesn't cause endorphin release (a possible reason for acupuncture's effectiveness). One theory is that hypnosis allows pain signals to be processed in the brain at an unconscious level; hypnosis prevents the signals from penetrating to the consciousness.

Advantages. Although hypnosis can provide long-lasting pain relief, it won't interfere with the patient's normal activities or incapacitate him mentally. And unlike many analgesics, hypnosis won't cause toxic effects, physical dependence, or tolerance.

Because hypnosis requires your patient's active participation, it usually changes his attitude toward his pain and his illness. It creates a sense of control in a chronic pain patient who may feel that he's a helpless victim of his pain. That feeling of control relieves the anxiety and hopelessness that can intensify his pain. For added effect, hypnosis can be coupled with such techniques as guided imagery.

Disadvantages. But hypnosis also has the following drawbacks:

- Because hypnosis must be conducted by a highly trained specialist, it can be expensive.
- During age regression (a hypnotic technique described on the following page), a patient may be faced with a traumatic event he can't cope with. This traumatic insight could trigger a full-blown psychosis in a susceptible patient.
- By making the patient feel better, hypnosis may cause him to ignore a real medical problem.
- Hypnosis can increase a patient's anxiety if the therapist unwittingly makes a suggestion that triggers a traumatic memory.
- The patient may become dependent on his therapist, believing that the therapist is responsible for relieving his pain.

Because of these disadvantages, hypnosis has failed to gain wide acceptance in the medical community. Some doctors feel uncomfortable using a treatment for which the mechanism of action is not understood. Others, believing that training the patient takes too much time, consider hypnosis impractical.

HYPNOSIS: FACT AND FICTION

For many people, the word *hypnosis* conjures up images of spinning gold watches and penetrating stares from mad scientists. Or they think of a parlor game that compels entranced victims to squawk like chickens. But all of these impressions are misleading. The following information will help you understand what hynotism is and how it can help your patients.

Fiction

Hypnosis puts a person to sleep.

Fact

Hypnosis is a state of heightened concentration. The subject's attention is so sharply focused that he ignores minor distractions.

Fiction

Hypnosis takes away a person's self-control, allowing the hypnotist to manipulate his behavior in any way imaginable.

Fact

Under hypnosis, no one can be forced to do anything he believes to be dangerous or immoral.

Fiction

Only the weak-willed or weak-minded can be hypnotized.

Fact

Research indicates that the ability to experience hypnosis is unrelated to intelligence, strength of character, or mental health. A skilled hypnotist can lead almost any consenting individual of normal intelligence into a hypnotic state, although some people respond more easily than others.

Fiction

A person must be coached into a hypnotic state; he is a passive participant in a process controlled by the hypnotist.

Fact

All hypnosis requires the subject's active cooperation. With practice, a person can evoke a hypnotic state by himself.

Fiction

A person can become so deeply hypnotized that he won't come out of the trance.

Fact

Hypnotized persons don't lose consciousness (as an anesthetized patient does), and they're in no danger of failing to wake up.

Fiction

Hypnosis can cure a disease or help a person solve a problem.

Fact

While it can create life-enhancing attitudes in a patient and relieve his anxiety, hypnosis can't cure diseases. However, it can change his perception of a problem.

HEAT AND COLD

HYPNOSIS TECHNIQUES FOR MANAGING PAIN

Although you won't teach hypnotic techniques, familiarize yourself with some of them so you can answer your patient's questions. *Note:* The choice of technique depends on the therapist, the patient, and the pain type.

• *Symptom suppression* blocks the patient's awareness of pain and helps him distance himself from his problem. Its effectiveness depends on the degree of pain and on the patient's ability to concentrate.

• *Symptom substitution* allows him to interpret his pain in a positive way. Instead of experiencing his sensation as pain, he feels a comfortable sensation such as pressure or warmth.

• *Moving the pain* to a smaller or less significant area of the body can allow a chronic pain patient to handle what was once unbearable. For example, a migraine sufferer might move pain from his head to his little finger.

• *Time distortion* capitalizes on a phenomenon we've all experienced: hours spent pleasantly seem to last only minutes; minutes spent in anguish seem to drag on forever. Under hypnosis, a patient can act on the suggestion that his painful episodes last only minutes while his pain-free times last hours.

• *Age regression* can help him discover the causes of his pain by letting him remember earlier traumatic events. Chronic pain that lasts an unreasonably long time after an injury may be linked to such earlier events. Once a patient confronts the memory, his pain may lessen or disappear.

• *Dissociation* may help when no other approach works. With this technique, the patient learns to separate himself from the painful body part.

HEAT: AN ANCIENT REMEDY

As evidenced by the Roman baths, Turkish steam rooms, and Japanese hot tubs, heat has long been recognized as a simple but effective pain-relief measure. No one knows exactly why, but these factors probably play a part:

• Because heat increases blood flow to injured tissues, it may relieve pain by removing the products of inflammation (such as histamine, bradykinin, and prostaglandins) that produce pain locally.

• It may help by stimulating nerve fibers that close the pain gate, preventing pain signals from traveling up the spinal cord to the brain. (For more on the gate control theory, see pages 16 and 17.)

• By promoting muscle relaxation, heat treatments can promote sleep and diminish tension and anxiety—all of which reduce pain.

Indications and precautions. Pain from bruises, muscle spasms, and arthritis typically responds well to heat treatment. But heat treatments aren't beneficial for all conditions. Heat won't relieve pain from scar tissue or from pressure on a nerve caused by a ruptured disc. Because heat dilates blood vessels and increases local blood flow, it's contraindicated after traumatic injuries when swelling and inflammation are present. It's also contraindicated for patients with clotting defects or with certain cancer types, because heat can stimulate cancer cell growth. *Important:* Use heat cautiously if your patient is severely depressed—it may intensify his depression.

Two heat therapy types. Chances are, you'll use superficial heat to manage your patient's pain. Deep-heat therapy is another option, but it requires special training and equipment. Here's how the two types compare:

Superficial heat. Using covered electric heating pads or heat lamps, you can apply dry heat directly to the skin over painful

CONTINUED ON PAGE 52

Applying deep and superficial heat

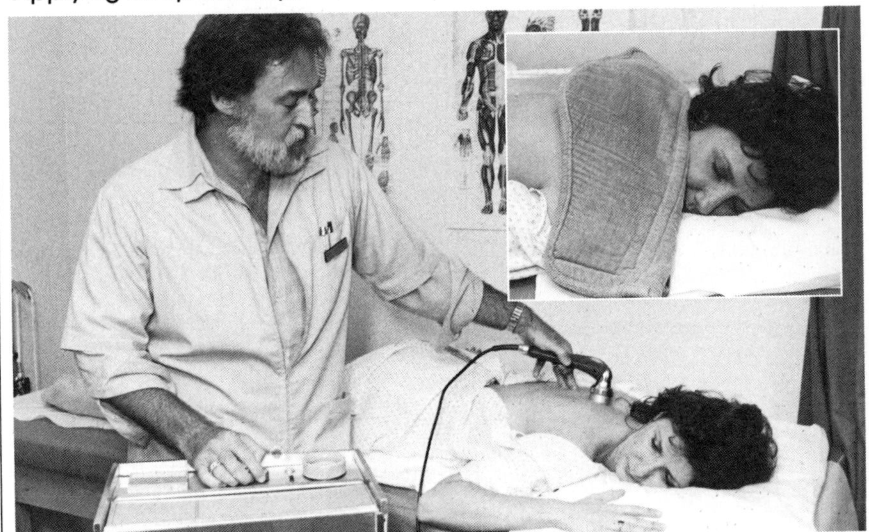

As shown above, a therapist can use an ultrasound device to provide deep-heat therapy for back pain. In the inset photo, the patient is undergoing superficial heat therapy with a hot pack.

HEAT AND COLD CONTINUED

HEAT: AN ANCIENT REMEDY CONTINUED

areas. To give a moist-heat treatment, use a hot pack, hot water bottle, or hot bath (such as a sitz bath for perineal pain). Or use a heating pad to apply moist heat by laying a moist towel over the painful area, covering it with a layer of insulation (for example, plastic wrap or a bedsaver pad) and laying the heating pad on top of the insulation. With this method, you can maintain continuous moist heat. *Caution:* Take care to check electric heating pads for frayed cords and other electrical hazards.

No matter what method you use, monitor the patient for burns. (Refer to the chart at right for temperature guidelines.) *Note:* Consider suggesting that your patient sit in the sun as a form of heat therapy. But advise him to avoid burning and apply a sunscreen.

Deep heat. Ultrasound and diathermy are two ways to apply heat to deep body structures, such as joints. With ultrasound, focused sound waves travel through soft tissue to solid structures, such as bone. There, they're absorbed and converted into heat. Diathermy, which heats painful deep structures with electromagnetic radiation, has largely been replaced by ultrasound as a deep-heating method.

Special Note:

To minimize the risk of causing a burn, use heat cautiously in areas of impaired sensation. Also use caution if the patient is sleepy or has a diminished level of consciousness; he may become burned without realizing it.

HEAT-THERAPY GUIDELINES

What's hot enough to help—without being *too* hot? Follow these guidelines. With the exception of hot compresses and hot soaks, continue heat therapy with each of these methods for 20 to 30 minutes or as ordered. Apply hot compresses for 15 to 20 minutes; hot soaks for 20 minutes.

HOT-WATER BOTTLE OR ELECTRIC HEATING PAD

For infants (to age 2) and geriatric patients: 105° to 115° F. (40.5° to 46.1° C.)
For other patients: 115° to 125° F. (46.1° to 51.6° C.)

INFRARED OR ULTRAVIOLET LIGHT

18″ to 24″ (45.7 to 70 cm) from the affected area (depending on equipment wattage)

GOOSENECK LAMP

At 25 watts: 14″ (35.5 cm) from the affected area

At 40 watts: 18″ (45.7 cm) from the affected area

At 60 watts: 24″ to 30″ (70 to 76 cm) from the affected area

AQUAMATIC K PAD

105° F. (40.5° C.)

HOT COMPRESS

131° F. (55° C.)

HOT SOAK

105° to 110° F. (40.5° to 43.3° C.)

COLD THERAPY: ANOTHER ALTERNATIVE

In contrast to heat therapy, which is effective for chronic pain, cold therapy is more effective for acute pain; for example, following soft-tissue injury from trauma, burns, cuts, or sprains.

Cold therapy works for several possible reasons:

- Cold slows the conduction velocity of nerves, reducing the number of pain impulses that reach the brain.
- Perceptual dominance of the cold sensation deadens the pain sensation.

Although speculative, another possible reason is that cold reduces inflammation (and, therefore, minimizes the amount of pain-producing substances released locally) by constricting peripheral blood vessels.

Some studies suggest that a combination of cold treatment and careful movement of injured areas considerably shortens post-trauma recovery time. Following orthopedic procedures, cold therapy can also reduce hemorrhage risk. Applied before a painful procedure such as I.M. injection or bone marrow aspiration, cold can deaden subsequent pain. Other painful conditions that respond well to cold therapy include headache and muscle spasm.

But cold therapy is contraindicated for patients with:

- history of allergic reaction (hives or joint pain) to cold therapy
- diabetes
- rheumatic disease (including arthritis)
- Raynaud's disease (cold may cause arterial spasm in the fingers and toes, reducing blood supply and risking gangrene).

Precautions. Remember that cold itself can cause an aching or burning pain; ice can cause burns. During cold therapy, monitor your patient closely for signs of discomfort.

Also, respect your patient's preferences regarding cold therapy. For example, although a substance such as Frigiderm can deaden sensation before an I.M. injection, many adult patients find the cold sensation more unpleasant than the injection pain. Many children, on the other hand, tolerate injections better after Frigiderm application.

If your patient is recovering from an injury, warn him that cold-induced numbness can be deceptive. Encourage him to move injured areas carefully and to avoid strenuous activity until healing is complete.

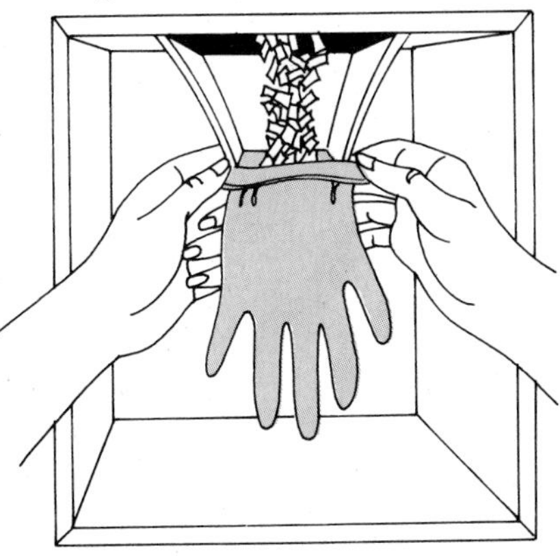

Ice therapy. Although Frigiderm, cold showers, and cold swims can benefit some patients, most cold therapy techniques require ice. Here are a few ways to apply ice therapy. *Note:* To reduce the risk of ice burns, consider applying oil to the patient's skin.

- An *ice towel* allows you to treat a large area, such as the lower back. Soak the towel in ice water (about 40° F. [4.4° C.]), wring it out, and place it directly on the painful area. Cover the towel with plastic wrap or a bedsaver pad, as insulation. When the towel becomes warm, resoak it.
- To give an *ice massage*, wrap a large chunk of ice in a washcloth and rub it on the painful area. Remove the ice after about 20 minutes. The patient may report that his skin no longer feels numb but is warm and tingling. Be careful not to leave the ice on too long; it can cause frostbite.
- You can use an *ice bath* to treat painful knees, ankles, elbows, and hands. Soak the injured part in 40° F. (4.4° C.) ice water for about 5 minutes; or hold it under cold water.
- In addition to relieving pain, an *ice pack* reduces swelling and bleeding. Make an ice pack by filling an ice bag, plastic bag, or disposable glove with ice.

Consider alternating heat therapy with cold therapy as a pain-control measure.

Ice bags have several disadvantages: In addition to being uncomfortably heavy, they may leak or slip out of place. Plastic bags and gloves are lighter and easier to prevent from leaking; chances are, they'll conform better to the area you're treating, too. (Other alternatives to ice bags are frozen gel packs or ice placed between towels.)

Wrap the ice pack in a towel, pillowcase, or washcloth, to protect the patient's skin from a burn. Adjust the intensity of cold by increasing or decreasing the number of cloth layers surrounding the ice pack, as needed.

Frequently check the ice pack and the patient's skin during treatment. As a rule, remove the ice within 20 minutes. Under some conditions, however, you can apply ice for longer periods; for example, when the affected area is in a cast.

COLD-THERAPY GUIDELINES

When using one of the methods listed below, follow these temperature guidelines.

ICE BAG

50° to 80° F. (10° to 26.6° C.) for 30 minutes

COLD COMPRESS OR PACK

59° F. (15° C.) for 15 to 20 minutes

CHEMICAL COLD PACK

50° to 80° F. (10° to 26.6° C.) for 30 minutes

COLD SOAK

59° F. (15° C.) for 20 minutes

AQUAMATIC K PAD

59° F. (15° C.) for 20 to 30 minutes

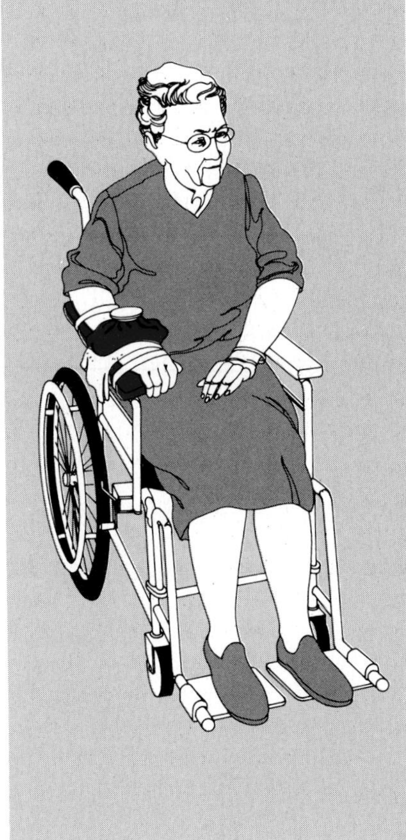

HEAT AND COLD CONTINUED

COMBINING COLD THERAPY AND CONTRALATERAL STIMULATION

If your patient's injury is too sensitive to be touched—or if you can't reach the injured area because of bandaging—you can still use cold therapy to relieve pain by applying ice to the opposite side of his body. Called *contralateral stimulation,* this technique works because impulses reaching the substantia gelatinosa in the spinal cord are influenced by sensory input from both sides of the body. As a result, pain-control measures applied to the contralateral (corresponding) body part may control pain on the affected side.

Contralateral cold stimulation can successfully control pain during such notoriously painful procedures as bone marrow aspiration. Because applying ice to the aspiration site would violate sterile technique, the patient massages the *contralateral* hip area with ice for 5 minutes. Then, the aspiration site is prepared and injected with a local anesthetic. After needle insertion—but before aspiration—the patient again massages the contralateral site with ice for about 1 minute. During bone marrow aspiration, he may feel little or no pain.

Note: Contralateral stimulation is also effective with other pain-control methods and devices, including transcutaneous electrical nerve stimulation (TENS). Similarly, a patient can relieve itching under a cast by scratching the contralateral body part.

Contralateral cold therapy before a painful procedure

By applying ice to the contralateral iliac crest, this patient minimizes the pain that will accompany bone marrow aspiration.

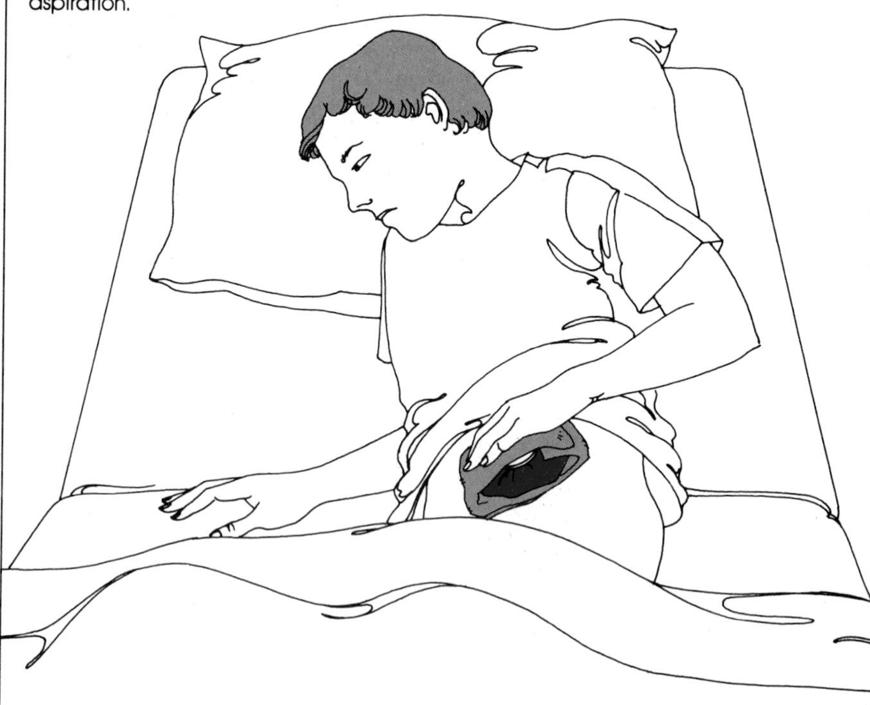

HOW MENTHOL RELIEVES PAIN

Menthol ointments, gels, creams, and liniments can relieve many pains, including the pain of arthritis and the muscle pain of sprains and spasms. Applied to the skin, menthol usually produces an almost immediate sensation of warmth, although some patients experience coolness.

How menthol ointments relieve pain remains a mystery. Methyl salicylate, an aspirin-like ingredient of most menthol ointments, may be responsible. Or menthol may stimulate the release of endogenous opioids such as endorphins. The placebo effect may also be a factor.

When you apply menthol ointments, you actually massage the patient's skin. That massage may itself contribute to menthol's pain-relieving effect: some patients derive relief and comfort from the touch. *Note:* A menthol massage can also be effective contralaterally.

Before you use menthol ointment on a patient, be sure to ask if he's allergic to menthol, finds the odor disagreeable (menthol has a strong and distinctive smell), or he dislikes the sensation of menthol on his skin. If he isn't allergic to menthol and doesn't object to this treatment, try applying a little menthol ointment on his skin near the painful area, to make sure it doesn't cause irritation. *Caution:* Never apply menthol ointment to broken or irritated skin or to mucous membranes.

If you find that menthol works for your patient, you can prolong his relief by using a plastic wrap or a bedsaver pad to insulate the menthol-coated area.

MASSAGE

MASSAGE: SIMPLE BUT EFFECTIVE

Massage is an instinctive response to pain. Picture yourself banging your elbow. Responding by reflex, you rub the site to ease the pain.

Why is massage so effective? According to the gate control theory, the action stimulates large-fiber nerve impulses, closing the pain gate. Other possible reasons for pain relief after massage include muscle relaxation and sedation.

Massage can be a useful strategy for treating patients with muscle aches, back pain, and neck pain. It can be done lightly or deeply, by either massaging the painful site itself or manipulating distant sites.

The back is ideal for massage because it's easily accessible. In addition, it includes many muscles that tire easily and become stressed. For many people, a back massage relieves tension in the entire body.

Other benefits. In addition to relieving pain, massage provides an opportunity for you to establish a rapport with your patient. Because massage requires touch, it's a direct form of nonverbal communication that suggests your concern for him. In addition, it lets you converse in a relaxed atmosphere and find out what's worrying him. By encouraging your patient to talk about his problems, you can help reduce the anxiety that exacerbates pain. During the massage, you also have a chance to look for pressure areas or dependent edema and to observe his general skin condition.

Basic principles. Although massage techniques differ in function and procedure, several principles guide all of them:

- Since each movement has a purpose, make each one slow and deliberate. Use firm, smooth, and even strokes; short, uneven strokes are uncomfortable.
- Be thorough. Use overlapping strokes to cover the entire area.
- When massaging arms and legs, always work toward the heart. When performed correctly, a massage not only improves venous return, it also promotes lymphatic drainage. *Caution:* Don't massage calf muscles if you know or suspect that the patient has thrombophlebitis.
- Be aware of both your own and your patient's breathing patterns. Exert more pressure when you exhale together.
- Remember that the patient's role is simply to relax and enjoy your massage. For details on several common massage techniques, see the information and photos beginning at right.

Myofascial release

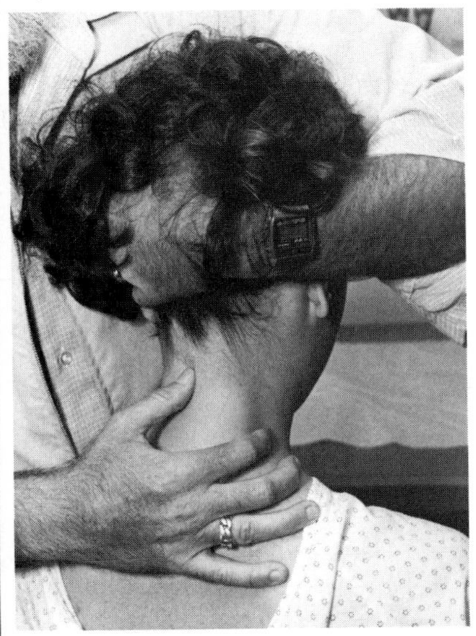

To perform this massage technique, a specially trained practitioner manipulates the fascia, a continuous, laminated sheet of connective tissue that extends from the top of the head to the tips of the toes. In theory, stretching this fascia promotes normal mobility, which in turn helps to prevent or relieve pain.

MASSAGE TECHNIQUES

The photos below and on the next page illustrate four basic massage techniques. The technique you choose depends in part on the desired effect. For example, petrissage and tapotement have a stimulating effect; effleurage has a relaxing effect.

Also consider your patient's condition and body structure. For example, avoid using tapotement on an emaciated patient; he'd probably find the technique uncomfortable. To use effleurage on an obese or muscular patient, however, you need to apply greater-than-usual pressure, to properly stimulate his muscles.

In the following photos, the nurse is demonstrating massage techniques on a patient's back. Note how he's positioned—prone, with his arms raised and his head turned to one side. If your patient can't assume this position, turn him to one side. Don't forget to raise the bed to a height that's comfortable for you.

CONTINUED ON PAGE 56

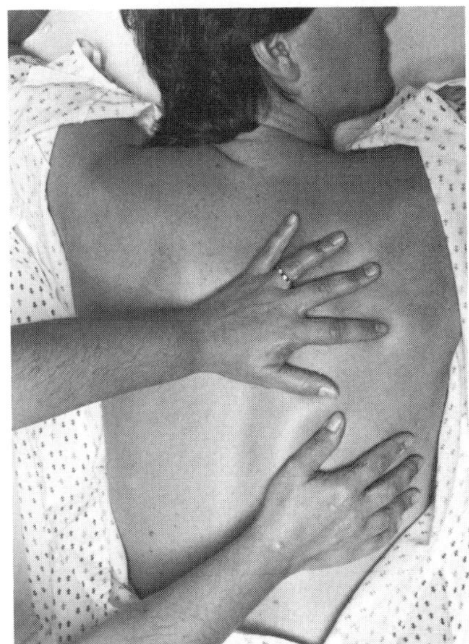

Effleurage: Using one or both thumbs or hands to make long, deep or superficial strokes.

MASSAGE CONTINUED

MASSAGE TECHNIQUES
CONTINUED

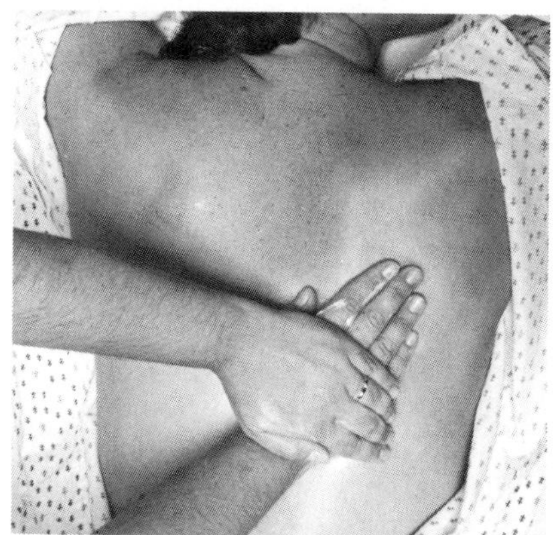

Petrissage: Placing one hand on the other to reinforce pressure and making circles or transverse strokes.

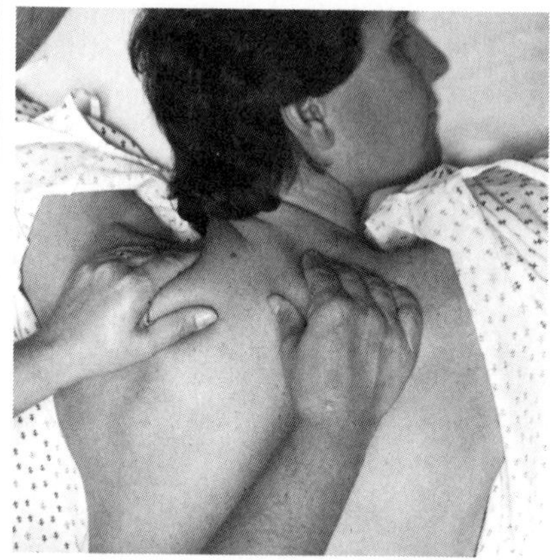

Kneading: Grasping a portion of a muscle group in each hand and gliding one hand toward the other as you squeeze.

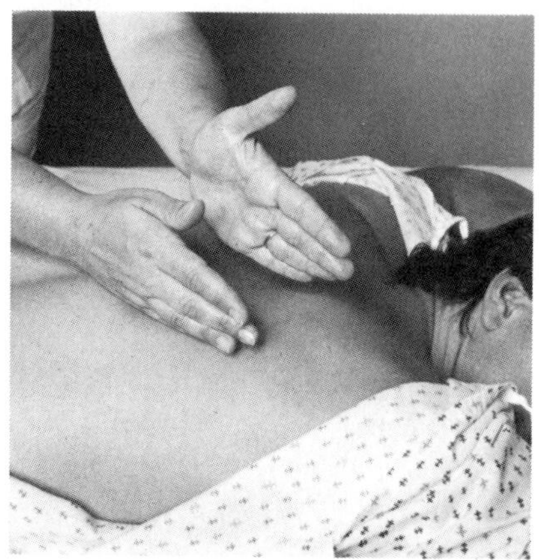

Tapotement: Using the hands in a chopping motion.

HOW TO GIVE A BENEFICIAL BACK RUB

Before giving a back rub, make sure you know your patient's diagnosis. A back rub is usually contraindicated for a patient with fractured ribs or for a patient who's recently had a heart attack or back surgery.

Preparation. Before starting, make sure your hands are warm and relaxed. Hold them under warm water or rub them together briskly. Since friction between your hands and the patient's back may cause irritation, use lotion or oil (for example olive or safflower oil) to lubricate his skin. Remember to warm the lotion or oil first, either in your hands or by placing the bottle in warm water. *Note:* Use alcohol followed by powder if your patient's skin is oily.

Plan a minimum of 4 minutes for a back rub; 6 minutes or more is even better.

The procedure. To begin the back rub, make contact with your patient by holding your hands on his back for a few seconds. Focus on the patient, even if he remains silent.

Starting at the base of the spine and using firm strokes, proceed upward to his shoulders. Rotate outward from his spine to include his entire back. Meanwhile, you may use the thumb and first three fingers of one hand to rub his shoulder or the nape of his neck.

Keeping both hands on the patient's back at all times, make smooth transitions as you move from one stroke to another. This is more comfortable and relaxing than if you were to remove your hands and reapply them during the back rub.

To end the back rub, use long strokes up the length of the patient's back, gradually reducing the pressure as you move your hands. These long, soothing strokes will further relax and comfort him.

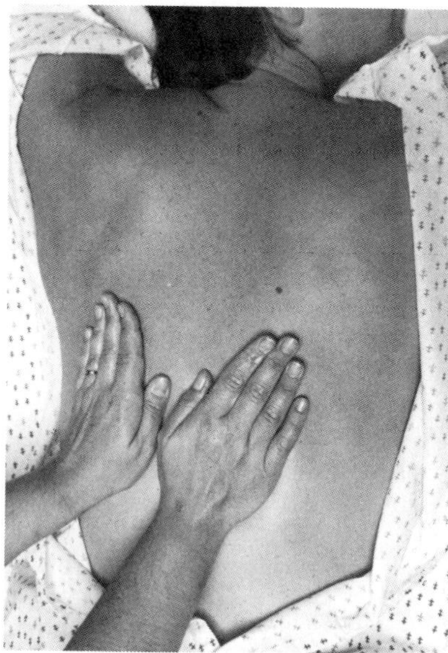

To begin a back rub, start at the base of the spine and work toward the shoulders.

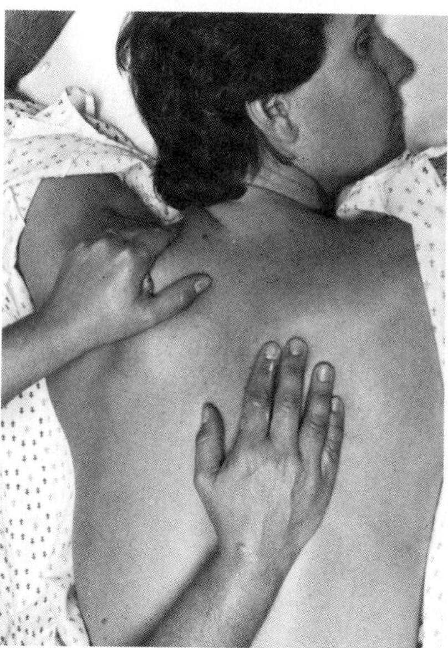

Use one hand to massage your patient's shoulder or neck while you continue the back rub with your other hand.

T.E.N.S.

RELIEVING PAIN WITH ELECTRICAL STIMULATION

Whether your patient has acute or chronic pain, he may respond to an increasingly popular pain-management device—the transcutaneous electrical nerve stimulator (TENS). A TENS unit consists of a battery-powered generator that sends a mild electrical current through electrodes placed on the skin at or near the pain site. The current produces a pleasant tingling or massaging sensation.

In addition to relieving pain, TENS increases blood flow near the electrodes, indirectly relaxing muscles and speeding the healing process. The patient can use TENS in the hospital, at home, or on the job.

Why does TENS work? No one knows for sure. According to one theory, TENS stimulates endorphin release. Another possible explanation, based on the gate control theory, is that electrical stimulation closes the gate to pain-impulse transmission.

Some TENS units, which are set at low frequency, work by stimulating muscle twitching and causing endorphin release. This TENS type is used primarily to treat pain related to muscle spasm.

The more common TENS type, set at high frequency, selectively stimulates A and C fibers, closing the pain gate. It's effective for both chronic and acute pain.

Indications. Although the typical TENS user has chronic back pain, TENS is also effective after knee, hip, or lower back surgery. But orthopedic patients aren't the only surgical patients who can benefit from TENS. *Any* patient with postoperative pain is a candidate for TENS use if narcotic drugs could impede his recovery, because TENS won't cause such drug-related adverse effects as respiratory depression.

To help the patient control postoperative pain, the doctor (or nurse) places the TENS electrodes on either side of the incision. He may do so during surgery or later in the patient's room.

Other indications for TENS use include phantom-limb pain, peripheral neuralgias, rheumatoid arthritis, and reflex sympathetic dystrophies.

TENS is particularly effective for treating acute, well-localized pain and for treating pain following cholecystectomy and thoracotomy.

Contraindications. Don't use TENS on a patient with a cardiac pacemaker because electrical current from the TENS unit could interfere with pacing. TENS is also contraindicated for patients with dysrhythmias. In addition, TENS' safety during pregnancy hasn't been established. (If your patient requires an EKG or continuous cardiac monitoring, be aware that the TENS current may interfere with accurate readings. If possible, have an R.F. filter installed to prevent artifact.)

Disadvantages. In addition to the equipment's expense, possible disadvantages include itching, skin irritation, and electrical burns from the unit's electrodes. However, a new self-adhering electrode reportedly avoids these problems.

If your patient develops skin irritation at the electrode sites, suggest that he substitute hand cream or hydrocortisone cream for the conductive jelly. Other possible solutions include using another brand of conductive jelly, changing the type of adhesive tape or electrode, and varying electrode positions.

Stimburst TENS unit

Designed for chronic pain patients, this lightweight unit can be attached to a belt or a waistband for use during daily activities.

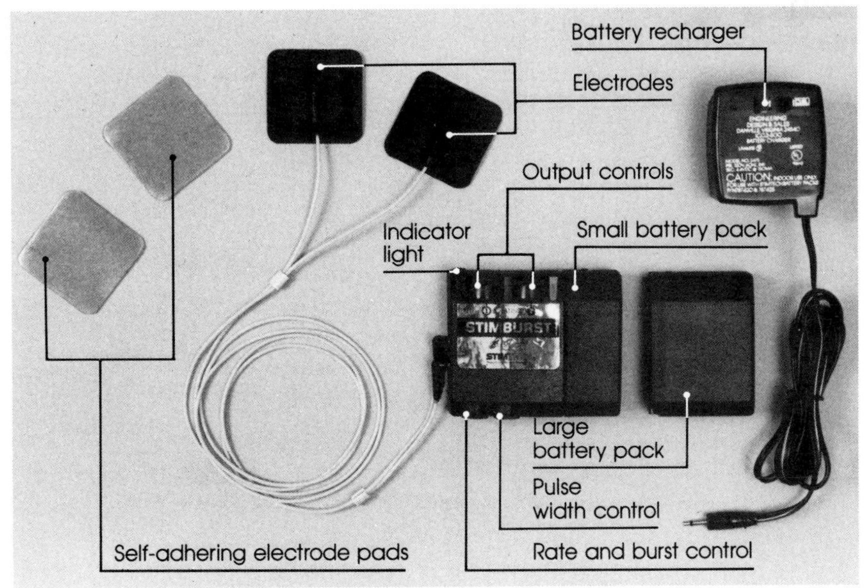

T.E.N.S. CONTINUED

A GUIDE TO T.E.N.S. USE

Before TENS therapy begins, make sure your patient understands how his TENS unit works, emphasizing that it may take a few days to find the most effective electrode placements and control settings. Explain that because pain relief may not be immediate, he should plan to use the TENS unit for at least a week before deciding if it helps.

Placing the electrodes. Electrode placement varies with each patient. Initially, the doctor, nurse, or TENS specialist may place the electrodes over an area where the nerve is relatively close to the skin's surface and thus more easily stimulated. For example, if your patient has pain in his arm, shoulder, or chest, the doctor may place the electrodes over the ulnar nerve at the elbow.

For radiating pain, he may position the electrodes over the nerve roots along the spine. To bombard a painful area such as the knee or lower back, he may place them in a crisscross pattern

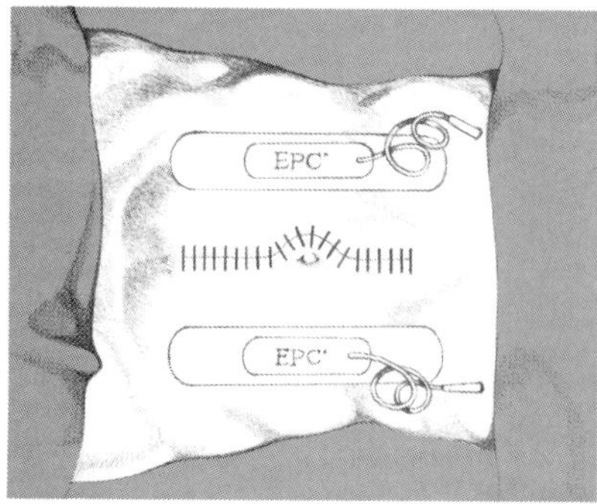

over that particular area. For postoperative pain, he'll probably place an electrode on either side of the incision, as shown above.

Placement of electrodes is crucial—a difference of $\frac{1}{16}$" (0.16 cm) can mean the difference between pain relief and increased pain. If the initial placement isn't effective, the doctor may choose a site closer to the painful area (for instance, along an involved nerve or near a painful scar) or along its dermatome. If this placement doesn't relieve the pain, he may try a location along the corresponding acupuncture meridian or muscle trigger point.

To apply TENS electrodes, follow these guidelines:

• Apply conductive jelly to each electrode. Use just enough to cover the electrode surface. (Self-adhering electrodes don't require

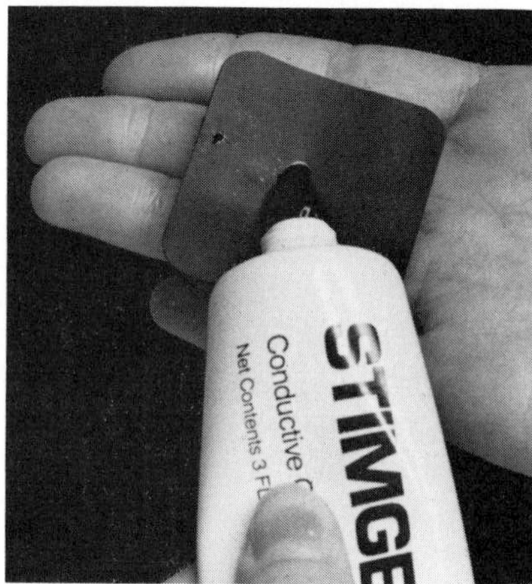

conductive jelly.)

• Position the electrodes so the distance between them is at least the width of an electrode—otherwise, your patient will be burned. Make sure each electrode is flat against the skin. *Caution:* Never place electrodes over laryngeal or pharyngeal muscles or over carotid sinus nerves. Also never place electrodes transcerebrally or on the eyes.

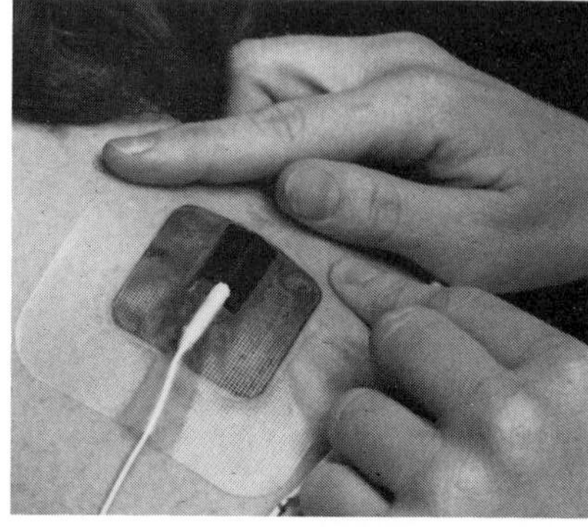

• Secure the electrodes. Use strips of tape that are just long enough to anchor the electrodes securely.

Adjusting the controls. All TENS units have dials or keys that control amplitude (intensity of stimulation) and pulse width (duration of each stimulation pulse). Some units have two channels, permitting the patient to use two electrode pairs simultaneously—either at the same pain site or at different sites. Each channel can be regulated separately.

The *amplitude* dial may be labeled *A* or *AMP* (for amplitude), *O* (for output, on, or off), *intensity,* or *energy.* (Some models have increase/decrease buttons and display amplitude readings on their digital display screens.) Although the dial may be calibrated from 1 to 5, 1 to 10, or 10 to 100, tell your patient to rely on feeling rather than numbers. He should feel a mildly or moderately pleasant sensation. A stimulation level that's too high may increase his pain and cause

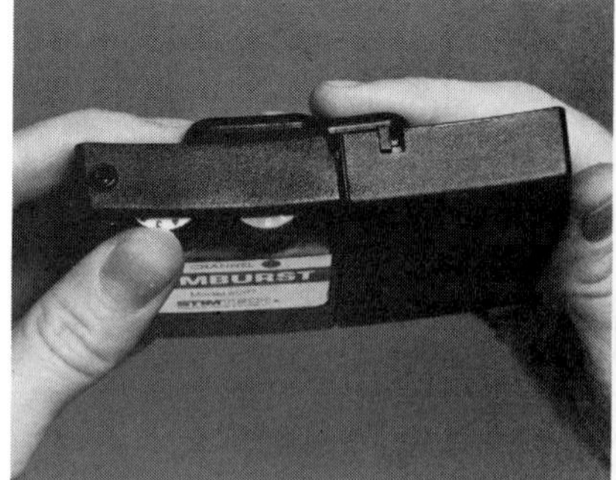

muscle spasms or itching.

The *rate* dial regulates the number of electrical impulses per second, ranging from 2 to 200 pulses. Although a high rate may relieve pain more quickly, warn the patient to increase the rate setting cautiously. If he feels an unpleasant sensation when turning up the rate, he should lower the amplitude or pulse-width dial.

The *pulse-width* dial determines the duration of each impulse, usually between 50 and 250 microseconds. (On some TENS units, pulse width is incorporated in the rate or amplitude dial.) In most cases, the patient should start with a lower pulse width when stimulating such small muscles as those in the back of the neck. For a patient with chronic pain, a mid-range pulse-width setting may deliver stimulation deep enough to relieve the pain without causing muscle spasms or itching.

TEACHING TIPS

Before your patient begins to use his TENS unit, teach him to:

- lock or tape the controls after setting them.
- remove the electrodes at least once a day (or as recommended) and clean the electrodes and his skin. If he's wearing his TENS continuously, he can then reapply the electrodes.
- remove the electrodes when he swims or takes a bath or shower. (Removing TENS at bedtime is also recommended; however, if your patient needs TENS to sleep, advise him to tape the electrodes and controls securely.)
- experiment with different control settings to learn which combination best relieves his pain. Tell him to record the combinations that work best. *Note:* Warn him against *excessive* voltage—higher voltage won't necessarily provide better pain relief.
- clean the unit regularly, using a damp cloth or sponge. To remove stains or adhesive on the stimulator case, tell him to use alcohol or a mild cleaning solution. Tell him not to immerse the unit in liquid.

EPC/Dual Electronic Pain Control Unit

This TENS unit, which includes sterile, self-adhering electrodes, is designed to control postoperative pain.

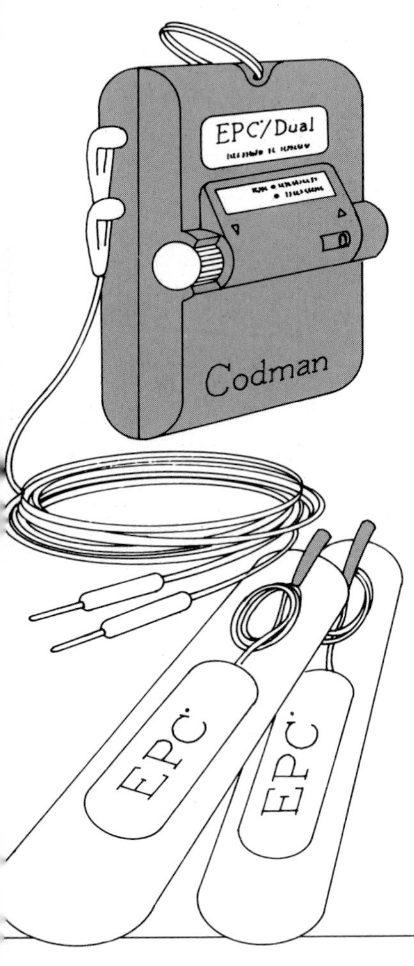

PERMANENT ELECTRICAL STIMULATION SYSTEMS

Some patients with chronic pain may benefit from a permanent implantable stimulation system. Like TENS, these systems interrupt pain pathways; however, they're much more powerful than TENS. Types of permanent electrical stimulation include dorsal column stimulation, peripheral nerve stimulation, and deep brain stimulation.

A similar but temporary type of electrical stimulation, percutaneous epidural dorsal column stimulation can be used to screen patients for possible permanent dorsal column stimulation. After the doctor implants wire electrodes in the spinal epidural space, the patient controls his own stimulation by adjusting the controls on an external battery-powered transmitter.

If percutaneous stimulation is successful, the doctor may recommend permanent *dorsal column stimulation.* If the patient agrees, the doctor performs a laminectomy in the high dorsal region, implants electrodes, and places the receiver in a subcutaneous pocket. The receiver is regulated by an externally worn transmitter.

Peripheral nerve stimulation may help a patient who has intractable pain associated with a specific peripheral nerve or nerve root. Electrodes implanted around the nerve are driven by a subcutaneous receiver, which in turn responds to signals from an external transmitter.

Deep brain stimulation alters the perception of pain by activating descending inhibitory pain messages from midbrain and brain stem structures. This method may work by stimulating endogenous opioid release, producing extremely potent analgesia.

Before implanting a permanent brain stimulator, the doctor inserts temporary electrodes. The patient then uses the temporary system for 10 days. If it relieves his pain, the doctor replaces the temporary electrodes with permanent ones.

Note: Although promising, the efficacy of permanent electrical stimulation is unproven; the procedure is still considered experimental.

BIOFEEDBACK

BIOFEEDBACK FACTS

Biofeedback provides a way for a patient to obtain previously unavailable information about specific body functions, such as his blood pressure or body temperature. By using this data, or feedback, he may then be able to modify certain physiologic functions; for example, his blood pressure or heart rate.

Major goals of biofeedback training include helping the patient learn to:

• become more aware of physiologic functions or events.

• establish control over these functions.

• continue this control, as needed, without the help of special equipment.

Why does biofeedback work? At one time, scientists believed that the autonomic nervous system alone controlled heart rate, blood pressure, blood flow, body temperature, and gastrointestinal motility. As a result, they presumed that these functions were unconscious, involuntary, and reflexive. Today we know this is not true. A patient can consciously control these activities to some extent, in many cases using biofeedback.

How does biofeedback work? During a biofeedback session, the therapist connects the patient to a machine that monitors physiologic functions; for example, body temperature (by skin sensors), muscle tension (by electromyography [EMG]), cardiovascular responses (by electrocardiography), or brain waves (by electroencephalography). Then, the therapist encourages the patient to relax, using whatever relaxation technique the patient prefers (for example, imagery or progressive muscle relaxation). The therapist will probably supply a relaxation tape as an aid. As the patient concentrates on relaxing, the equipment provides constant feedback in the form of audible tones, lights, or digital readings.

Feedback is based on physiologic changes that reflect relaxation; for example, a temperature change in the hands. Why is hand temperature a good indicator? Because as the patient relaxes, sympathetic nervous system activity diminishes and vessels dilate. As peripheral blood supply improves, the hands become warmer.

As a result of this feedback, the patient knows immediately when he begins to relax. He can then determine which images, thoughts, and other cognitive strategies work best for him.

Who can biofeedback help? Biofeedback training can be especially helpful for controlling the pain of muscle tension and stress, including lower back pain and headaches. With headache patients, biofeedback works best for those who experience such prodromes as the bright, flashing lights that sometimes precede migraine headaches. This physiologic warning provides the patient with a chance to ward off his headache before it's a reality.

Biofeedback can also control essential hypertension; regulate blood flow (as in Raynaud's disease); help control cardiac dysrhythmias; retrain muscles in patients with hemiplegia, spasticity, and paralysis; and relieve insomnia and anxiety-related syndromes.

WEIGHING ADVANTAGES AND DISADVANTAGES

Why might the doctor recommend biofeedback to your patient in pain? For starters, biofeedback helps the patient participate in his treatment. By providing immediate feedback, it gives the patient a sense of control and accomplishment. In contrast, a more traditional treatment, such as drug therapy, encourages the patient to play a passive role and diminishes his sense of control over his condition.

If the patient's taking analgesics, biofeedback can have an additional benefit: it may allow the doctor to reduce the dosage as the patient learns to effectively manage his pain.

Biofeedback is noninvasive and virtually risk-free. Furthermore, it's proven effective for many patients in pain. But what about the disadvantages? Consider the following points:

• Learning biofeedback techniques requires a specially trained therapist and special equipment.

• Training is time-consuming because treatment must be individualized and the patient must practice regularly to achieve results. For example, he may need to practice with the special equipment for 20 minutes, one to three times weekly. In addition, he must practice without the equipment several times every day.

• The patient must be highly motivated to learn the techniques and willing to wait several months or more for results.

Biofeedback isn't for everyone; it requires the patient's special interest and enthusiasm. If your patient's reluctant or passive, he may respond better to some other therapy.

YOUR ROLE

Although you won't teach your patient biofeedback techniques, you may be responsible for preparing her to begin a training program and for answering her questions.

First, familiarize her with biofeedback, and discuss its pros and cons. Explain that the long-range goal of therapy is for her to learn to achieve effective pain control without using special equipment. *Note:* Make sure she doesn't harbor misconceptions about the therapy or equipment; for example, she may think that the equipment will give her a shock.

Also, tell her what she should expect during a training session. Although training techniques and equipment vary among clinics, a typical session proceeds as follows.

The therapist takes the patient into a quiet room and seats her in a comfortable chair. He then places electrodes on her forehead, explaining that they will measure forehead muscle tension because it reflects tension in the rest of the body. The higher the tone emitted from the biofeedback machine, the higher the level of registered tension. To measure skin temperature, he also places electrodes on her hand.

The therapist then leads the patient through a progressive muscle relaxation session. His goal is to have her decrease the machine's warning tone by relaxing.

At the end of the session, he evaluates how the therapy proceeded and teaches the patient how to use the technique at home. He emphasizes that good results are possible only with diligent practice.

Special Note:

In most cases, the therapist records training exercises, along with detailed instructions, on cassette tapes so the patient can use them at home. Home practice cassettes of this kind help decrease the patient's dependence on biofeedback equipment.

Using biofeedback for pain control

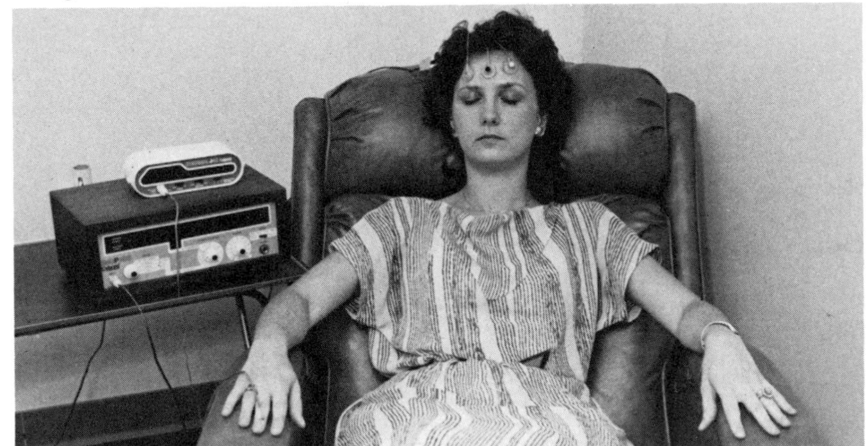

During this biofeedback session, the patient is learning to raise skin temperature and lower pulse rate and muscle activity. The log below traces her progress.

Biofeedback Log

Name: Joan Sandell

Type of pain: Low back pain

Brief history: Fell off a ladder at home 1 year ago. Has been treated with bed rest, analgesics and physical therapy without relief. Referred for comprehensive evaluation, including biofeedback training.

Date	Parameters fed back	Parameters monitored	Goal	Goal achieved Yes/No	Response to treatment (see key)	Comments and signature
9/25	Skin temperature pulse rate	Skin temperature pulse rate	↑ temp by 5 °F ↓ pulse by 5 beats per minute ↓ EMG reading	yes	NC	This is the first session patient told that pain relief may not occur initially. Patient to return on 9/27. Relaxation tape given and patient instructed in its use. M. Motah R.P.T.

KEY: W = Worse, **NC** = No change, **SI** = Some improvement, **PR** = Pain relief

ACUPUNCTURE

MODERN USES FOR AN ANCIENT REMEDY

Although acupuncture dates back thousands of years, many people view this ancient Chinese pain-relief technique with skepticism. But because recent research suggests a scientific basis for acupuncture (see box below), it's becoming more widely accepted among Western health-care professionals as an alternative to analgesic and anesthetic drugs for some patients.

Licensing requirements for acupuncture practitioners vary throughout the United States and Canada. Because needle acupuncture is an invasive procedure that carries a slight risk of infection or damage to nerves and blood vessels, some states require that the practitioner be a medical doctor.

Note: Not all acupuncture techniques are invasive. For details, see page 63.

The procedure. To perform traditional acupuncture, the practitioner inserts long, extremely thin needles into specific acupuncture (or hoku) points located along a series of channels called meridians. Each meridian runs along a major body part and ends at the fingertips or toes.

Practitioners have identified (by name and number) about 1,000 acupuncture points, each about ⅛″ (0.25 cm) in diameter. Most points belong to one of 14 groups associated with internal organs.

To select appropriate acupuncture points, the practitioner first takes a detailed patient history. He may then use traditional Chinese diagnostic techniques to obtain more information.

To treat the patient's disease or injury, the practitioner may need to stimulate several acupuncture points. For a typical treatment, he inserts 10 to 15 needles at varying angles and depths. (Unlike hypodermic needles, acupuncture needles have rounded tips that push tissue aside without cutting it.)

After insertion, the practitioner may twist or vibrate the needles (either manually or electrically) to maximize stimulation. Or he may heat the needles with burning herbs (moxa). The length of time for each treatment varies, according to the intended result.

Patient response. During treatment, the patient may feel sensations ranging from pin pricks, warmth, light-headedness, or heaviness to stinging or a dull, aching throb. The practitioner then increases stimulation at certain acupuncture points. As treatment progresses, the patient will be able to tolerate more stimulation, although he may feel some discomfort during treatment.

The patient may get relief from his pain immediately after the first treatment. Or he may require as many as 20 treatments before feeling significant relief. *Note:* Some patients never respond to treatment.

Some acupuncture points on the back of the right hand

This key identifies the acupuncture points shown in the illustration below.

1 Waist and leg
2 Spine
3 Occipital lobe
4 Perineum
5 Temporal lobe
6 Frontal lobe
7 Throat
8 Sciatic nerve
9 Neck
10 Eye
11 Shoulder

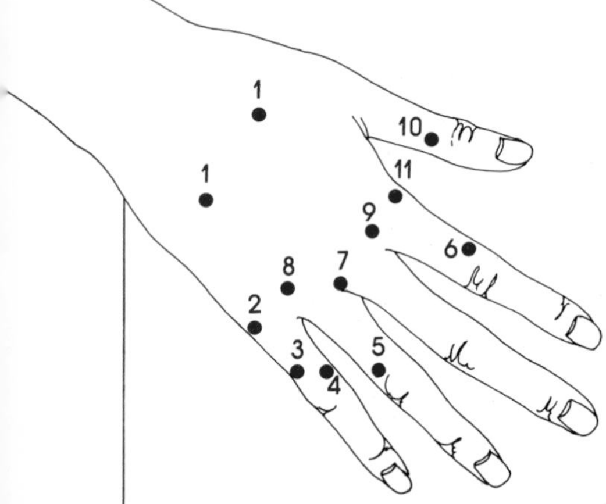

WHY ACUPUNCTURE WORKS: TRADITIONAL AND SCIENTIFIC THEORIES

Why does acupuncture provide pain relief? The Chinese answer this question in terms of Yin and Yang, two universal life forces represented in the body by spirit and blood, respectively. According to this theory, each force moves along the meridians. Pain and illness develop when Yin and Yang fall out of harmony. Insertion of acupuncture needles at specific points allows Yin and Yang to reestablish harmony.

Searching for a more scientific explanation, Western researchers have developed several alternative theories. One explanation, based on the gate control theory, is that acupuncture stimulates the larger sensory nerve fibers that carry nonpain impulses. At the spinal level, these impulses inhibit pain conduction from smaller fibers—closing the pain gate.

Another possible explanation is that acupuncture triggers release of endorphins and other endogenous opioids, producing analgesia. This theory is supported by the apparent fact that administration of a morphine antagonist such as naloxone reverses acupuncture's analgesic effects. *Note:* Some studies have failed to confirm this phenomenon.

USES FOR ACUPUNCTURE

Acupuncture may be effective for such disorders as:
- headache
- musculoskeletal pain
- premenstrual or menstrual pain
- stress, tension, and nervousness
- some neuralgias
- hypertension
- lower back pain
- insomnia
- dental and facial pain.

Acupuncture has also helped some patients to lose weight and others to stop smoking.

Surgery. Chinese doctors report that acupuncture produces such profound analgesia that major surgery can be performed without an additional anesthetic—while the patient is fully conscious. In the West, acupuncture's value as a surgical anesthetic isn't established. Should acupuncture anesthesia become accepted, however, it offers these advantages:
- It won't lower blood pressure or depress respirations.
- The patient may lose less blood during surgery, according to some studies.
- The patient won't suffer anesthesia-related postoperative adverse effects.
- Because analgesic effects persist for several hours, the patient needs less postoperative pain medication.

In some cases—for example, surgery to correct strabismus—the patient's ability to cooperate is another advantage.

Disadvantages. As a treatment for chronic pain, acupuncture has several drawbacks. Because the patient may need many sessions with a specially trained practitioner, treatment can be expensive. And he can't rely on acupuncture to relieve pain between treatments. Perhaps most important, studies haven't established lasting benefits for chronic pain patients.

NONINVASIVE ACUPUNCTURE TYPES

Acupressure, electronic acupuncture, and cold laser therapy use traditional acupuncture points and meridians to relieve pain. Unlike traditional acupuncture, however, these techniques are noninvasive. Here's how they compare.

Acupressure. Instead of using needles, the practitioner stimulates acupuncture points by pressing, rubbing, or pounding them with his thumbs. The patient can learn to perform this technique himself.

Electronic acupuncture. To use this technique, which is similar to TENS, the practitioner stimulates acupuncture points with a special electronic device called a neuroprobe. He gradually increases the strength and intensity of the stimulation to the patient's level of tolerance. As treatment progresses, the patient can tolerate more stimulation with less discomfort.

Cold laser therapy. Compared to acupuncture, which can produce quick but short-lived pain relief, cold laser therapy has long-term effects. As a result, it's often used with acupuncture. Unlike hot laser beams used for microsurgery, cold laser beams don't damage tissue.

For pain-relief therapy, the practitioner applies conductive jelly to an acupuncture point. Then, he positions the laser tube's tip directly on the patient's skin. During therapy, the patient may feel either a slight tingle or no sensation at all. *Note:* The practitioner can also direct the beam into a painful joint or other body part.

Although speculative, possible explanations for cold laser therapy's effectiveness include the following:
- According to the *bioluminescence* theory, a disease or other abnormal condition diminishes the normal energy level of tissue cells. The laser beam may help restore normal energy levels.
- Nerve tissues may transmit laser energy in much the same way optic fibers do, explaining the laser's beneficial effects on distant body parts.
- The laser may trigger release of endogenous opioids.

Cold laser therapy is contraindicated during pregnancy. Also, the laser beam should never be directed into a patient's eye, although he may safely view the beam indirectly.

Electronic acupuncture

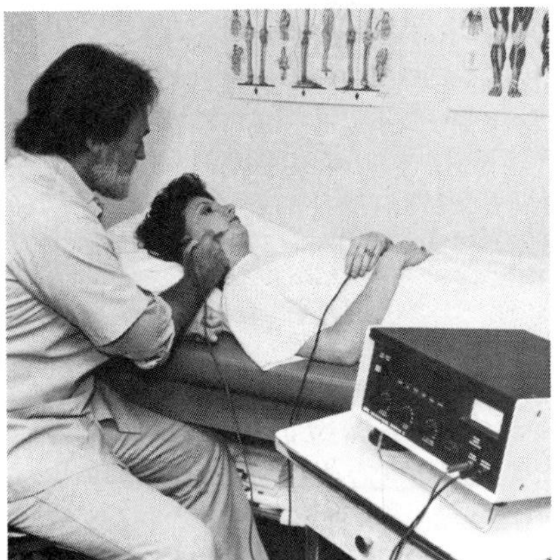

During both of these noninvasive acupuncture procedures, the patient holds a ground wire.

Cold laser therapy

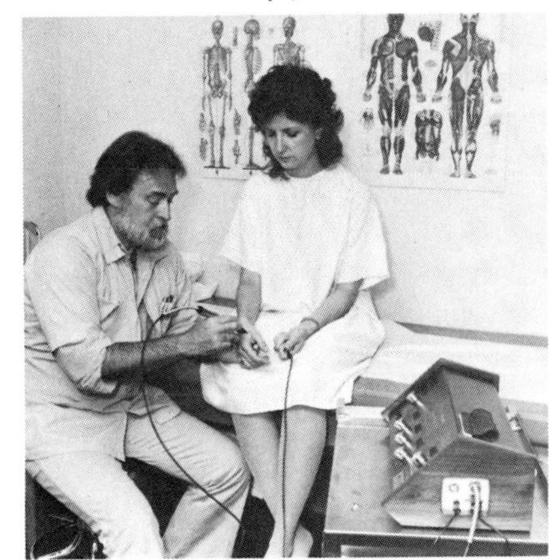

ALTERNATIVE THERAPIES

CHANGING PAIN BEHAVIOR

You can help some of your patients manage their pain with behavior modification, a technique designed to systematically encourage desirable behavior and discourage undesirable behavior.

A chronic pain patient may be accustomed to receiving attention for such undesirable pain behaviors as moaning and withdrawing. By discouraging these behaviors and rewarding healthier behaviors with the constructive use of attention and approval, you can help him resume a more normal life-style.

Getting started. Although behavior modification is best suited for pain clinics, you can incorporate elements of it into your care plan. Follow these steps:

• *Perform an assessment.* Identify inappropriate behaviors, and determine how frequently these behaviors occur. With pain patients, particularly those in chronic pain, these behaviors typically include physical inactivity, decreased sexual activity, aggressiveness or anger, frequent complaints about pain, diminished appetite, depression, and withdrawal from family and friends.

• *Set goals.* At this stage, you must involve the patient, his family and friends, and the health-care team. Help the patient define goals to be reached within a specified time period. Initially, his goals should be easily attainable, to prevent him from becoming discouraged.

Suppose, for example, that Mr. Matthews is unwittingly isolating himself from others with his incessant complaints about pain. Discuss his behavior—and how to change it—with him and his family. Mr. Matthews might agree to try for these two goals: to minimize his complaints and to increase his activity by walking down the hall twice a day.

• *Delineate the reinforcers.* You and your patient should agree on whether to use positive reinforcement, negative reinforcement, or both. The reinforcers you choose will depend on your patient's behavior and preferences. However, most patients respond better to such positive reinforcers as attention, affection, and approval.

Behavior modification depends on the cooperation of everyone involved, especially family members.

If your patient's goal is to walk down the hall twice a day, for example, positive reinforcers could be attention and approval lavished by you and his family after each walk.

As a negative reinforcer, you could respond to a pain complaint by saying, "Mr. Matthews, we agreed we weren't going to talk about your pain so much. I'm going to leave now—I'll be back in 10 minutes." Then, leave.

Reinforcement can be either continuous (reinforcing every correct response) or intermittent (reinforcing only some correct responses). Learning is faster with continuous reinforcement. However, you may find that the best strategy is to use continuous reinforcement for teaching the desired behavior and then gradually switching to intermittent reinforcement to maintain the target behavior.

Program assessment. Evaluate your program's success after it's been in effect for a predetermined length of time. If you and your patient haven't achieved the goals, revise the program and try again.

EXPLORING OTHER PAIN-RELIEF OPTIONS

Still considered faddish by mos members of the medical comm nity, a number of unconvention pain-relief therapies have become increasingly popular among some chronic pain suffe ers. Although some of these therapies have been partially validated by scientific research, others remain unsubstantiated.

Why, then, do these therapie continue to attract patients? Th simple answer is that, while the reasons may be unclear, they have helped some chronic pain sufferers who haven't had success with conventional medical therapy.

If your patient asks you abou an unconventional therapy, you should know enough about it to answer his questions and provi guidance—regardless of your personal opinions about it. Remember, even the possibility of pain relief—however slim—can mean the difference between hope and despair.

First, find out what he knows about the therapy he's consider ing. Then, advise him to check with his doctor before beginnin any type of alternative therapy. Use the following information as a guide during patient teaching.

Chiropractic. Still unrecognized by the American Medical Assoc ation, chiropractic is a widely used therapy with a fairly simp theoretical basis. According to chiropractic theory, illness and pain occur when a person's vertebrae are out of alignment. By using physical manipulation to realign them, a chiropractor attempts to cure disease and elim nate pain.

Caution a patient considering chiropractic to have a medical doctor carefully evaluate his pai first, to determine if other forms of therapy are indicated and to rule out spinal conditions that could be exacerbated by manipulation.

Orgone therapy. Like chiropractic, orgone therapy involves physical manipulation. Unlike chiropractic, however, orgone therapy is based on the assumption that thoughts and emotions are simultaneously reflected in the body. Theoretically, neurotic psychological traits contribute to distinct, rigid physical traits that lead to illness and pain.

One type of orgone therapy, *bioenergetics*, employs stretching, breathing exercises, and deep massage to release tension, increase vitality, and encourage spontaneous emotional responses. According to one report, bioenergetics has been successful in relieving chronic tension headaches.

Rolfing. Practitioners of this technique attempt to relieve muscle tension and realign body weight with rigorous physical manipulations and deep-tissue massage. The goal is to help the patient move more naturally with gravity and so experience less pain.

Most rolfing practitioners schedule about 10 weekly 1-hour sessions. Tell the patient that, because the practitioner applies considerable force and pressure, rolfing can be painful. However, pain relief should follow the procedure.

Therapeutic touch. This ancient practice is based on the assumption that each person has energy fields that change when he becomes ill. The practitioner searches for a change in the patient's energy field—pain, for instance, feels hot and tight—and attempts to correct it by transmitting his own healing energy to the patient.

The procedure consists of two steps: First, the practitioner meditates to quiet his mental, emotional, and physical energies and to form the intention of transmitting energy to the patient. Then, he uses both hands to locate the painful area and transmit his healing energy.

Although a scientific basis for therapeutic touch hasn't been established, possible reasons for its effectiveness in some cases include the following:

- The laying on of hands may stimulate neural receptors in the skin at traditional acupuncture points.
- It may trigger the placebo response.
- It may stimulate the patient's emotional sense of well-being through physical contact with the practitioner.

Faith healing. No one knows exactly how faith healing works. One theory purports that it produces the placebo effect. By appealing to a patient's emotions and reducing his fears and anxieties, faith healing may also instill a positive, hopeful attitude. In the process, the patient's normal healing powers may be potentiated.

Tryptophan supplements. Some advocates of vitamin and nutrition therapy recommend supplements of tryptophan, an essential amino acid, taken along with such vitamins as niacin and B_6. How can tryptophan relieve pain? In the body, it's converted into serotonin, a neurotransmitter that potentiates morphine analgesia and suppresses pain at the central level. Tryptophan may also alleviate such pain-related symptoms as depression and insomnia.

Foods high in tryptophan include eggs, bananas, milk, and leafy green vegetables. But because these foods contain other amino acids that compete with tryptophan for transport mechanisms, dietary intake may not be adequate for pain relief. To raise levels of tryptophan and serotonin in the brain, the patient may be advised to eat a low-protein, high-carbohydrate diet and to take 2 to 4 g of tryptophan supplements per day.

One type of therapeutic touch

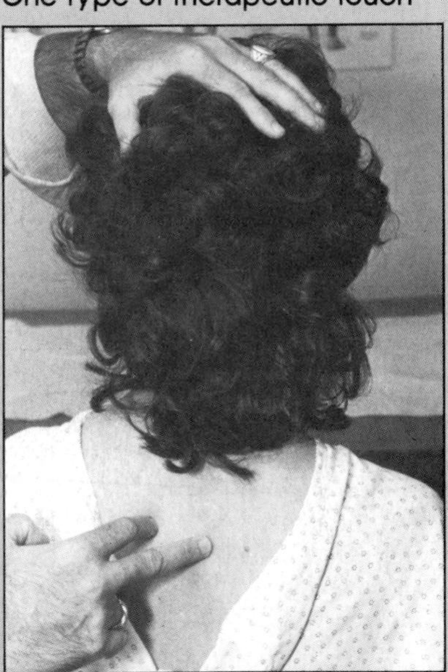

In this photo, the practitioner attempts to relieve neck pain with a therapeutic touch technique.

NERVE BLOCKS

BLOCKING PAIN

Many patients are familiar with nerve blocks as a short-term pain-relief measure—by injecting lidocaine into the gums, dentists routinely use nerve blocks to prevent pain during dental procedures. Although especially effective for treating acute pain, nerve blocks also have diagnostic and therapeutic value for treating chronic pain.

How they work. Most nerve blocks are achieved by injecting a local anesthetic into or around a peripheral nerve, into the spine, or into a major nerve plexus. Doing so inhibits pain-impulse conduction and provides local pain relief lasting 4 to 8 hours in most cases. Neurolytic nerve blocks, however, can provide long-term relief by permanently damaging nerve pathways.

Nerve block types. A *diagnostic* block is performed with a local anesthetic. It helps the doctor identify pain pathways and specific structures involved in the patient's pain. It can also help him separate and evaluate the physical and emotional components of the patient's pain.

Most *therapeutic* blocks provide short-term pain relief from such acute conditions as pancreatitis, costochondritis, and renal colic that may respond poorly to narcotic analgesics and other pain-relief measures. Although providing immediate pain relief, a single therapeutic block rarely relieves pain for more than 8 hours. However, for some patients—for example, those with musculoskeletal pain—repeated nerve blocks can produce progressively longer periods of pain relief. In some cases, pain relief lasts for months or even years.

Unlike other therapeutic blocks, which involve injection of a local anesthetic, neurolytic blocks are achieved by injection of a caustic agent—alcohol or phenol—into the subarachnoid space or into the affected nerve, destroying nerve tissue. An extreme measure, neurolytic blocks can lead to numbness or a painful inflammatory response that may be worse than the original complaint.

Prognostic blocks help the doctor determine the probable effect of a neurolytic block or a surgical procedure to destroy nerve pathways. Because the prognostic block can produce the same adverse effects as these procedures, the doctor and the patient can weigh the likely benefits against probable adverse effects before deciding on an irreversible procedure.

YOUR ROLE DURING A NERVE BLOCK PROCEDURE

Is your patient scheduled for a nerve block? Make sure you know your responsibilities by reviewing these guidelines:

- Obtain a pain history. Even if you can't do a complete patient assessment, you still should check your patient's history and recent laboratory test results for blood dyscrasias, neurologic disease, and major circulatory disturbances.
- Instruct the patient to avoid sudden movements during the procedure, and reassure him that discomfort will be minimal. Make sure he knows which adverse effects to report.
- Make sure the doctor obtains written consent.
- Check all equipment.
- During the procedure, provide the patient with ongoing support.
- During and after the procedure, closely observe him for complications. Tell him to report any unusual sensations below the block.

HOW TO RECOGNIZE AND MANAGE NERVE BLOCK COMPLICATIONS

Use this chart as a guide to possible postprocedure adverse effects.

SYSTEMIC REACTION TO LOCAL ANESTHETIC

Signs and symptoms

Mild reaction: Dysarthria, lightheadedness, vertigo, headache, apprehension, tachycardia, slight hypertension, and mouth dryness

Moderate reaction: Confusion, muscle twitching (usually progressing to convulsions), hypertension, and tachycardia

Severe reaction: Loss of consciousness, coma, severe hypertension, bradycardia, and respiratory depression

Nursing management

- *Mild reaction:* Reassure the patient and provide emotional support.
- *Moderate reaction:* Closely monitor the patient and be prepared for emergency intervention if symptoms progress.
- *Severe reaction:* Assist with intubation and cardiopulmonary resuscitation.

SUBARACHNOID BLOCK (FROM INADVERTENT INJECTION OF LOCAL ANESTHETIC INTO THE SUBARACHNOID SPACE)

Signs and symptoms

Respiratory weakness or paralysis

Nursing management

- Provide immediate respiratory support.
- Prepare to help the doctor aspirate 10 to 15 ml of spinal fluid, to reduce the amount of anesthetic in the subarachnoid space.
- Support circulation with fluids or vasopressors, as ordered.

HYPOTENSION (ASSOCIATED WITH CELIAC PLEXUS BLOCK)

Signs and symptoms
Sudden drop in blood pressure

Nursing management
- Administer I.V. fluids, as ordered.
- Give vasopressors, as ordered.

HEMATOMA

Signs and symptoms
Discoloration, swelling, and possible bleeding at the injection site

Nursing management
- Apply cold packs and pressure to the injection site.
- Monitor hemoglobin and hematocrit values; be prepared to transfuse blood products, if ordered.

PNEUMOTHORAX (ASSOCIATED WITH A PARAVERTEBRAL, STELLATE GANGLION, BRACHIAL OR CERVICAL PLEXUS, OR SPLANCHNIC NERVE BLOCK)

Signs and symptoms
Tachypnea, shortness of breath, restlessness, and other signs of respiratory distress

Nursing management
- Assist with chest-tube insertion, as ordered.
- Obtain a chest X-ray, as ordered.

SURGERY

NEUROSURGICAL INTERVENTIONS

As we learn more about pain mechanisms, we move closer to unraveling the complexities of pain pathways.

For years, traditional neurosurgical procedures focused on transecting a peripheral nerve, nerve root, or central tract. But time and experience have proven that this approach rarely achieves long-term pain relief; in fact, it may cause pain to worsen or cause new pain.

Today, however, neurosurgical pain-relieving procedures focus on interrupting pain pathways at three major levels—the peripheral level (first-order neurons), the spinal level (second-order neurons), and the brain level (third-order neurons).

A cordotomy, which interrupts pain transmission at the level of second-order neurons, is performed on the side contralateral (opposite) to the painful body part.

How do these neurosurgical procedures work? Let's consider the peripheral level first. First-order neurons transmit pain impulses from the receptor, along the peripheral nerve, and into the dorsal horn. Procedures such as nerve block, neurectomy, sympathectomy, and rhizotomy interrupt pain pathways at the level of first-order neurons.

Within the dorsal horn, first-order neurons synapse with second-order neurons. Second-order neurons send axons to the other side of the spinal cord; as a result, pain impulses ascend to the thalamus along the lateral spinothalamic tract on the opposite side. A cordotomy interrupts the lateral spinothalamic tract at the level of second-order neurons.

In the thalamus, second-order neurons synapse with third-order neurons. These sensory neurons transmit pain impulses to the cerebral cortex, where pain perception occurs. Stereotactic placement of surgical lesions and stimulating electrodes in the thalamus may interrupt pain pathways at the level of third-order neurons.

"Surgical procedures should be undertaken only if they are well conceived and well planned. The three surgical procedures that are most useful and that have demonstrated efficacy are cordotomy for unilateral pain below the waist; hypophysectomy for metastatic bone pain (particularly from hormonally sensitive tumors); and sympathectomy, either chemical or surgical, for the relief of causalgic pain syndromes."

Richard Payne, MD
Assistant Attending Neurologist
Memorial Sloan-Kettering
Cancer Center
New York

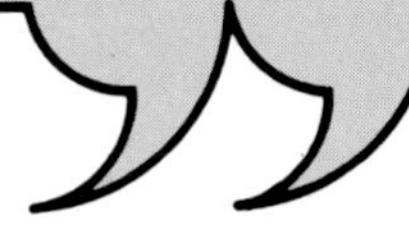

SURGERY CONTINUED

NURSE'S GUIDE TO NEUROSURGICAL PAIN-RELIEF PROCEDURES

No one neurosurgical procedure successfully relieves all types of pain. For this reason, you must be familiar with all the surgical options available to a patient in pain, including their expected benefits and risks. The first three procedures listed below are generally considered the most effective; the remaining procedures are infrequently performed.

For some neurosurgical pain procedures, the doctor uses stereotactic techniques. After locating internal brain landmarks, he produces small brain lesions with a cryosurgical probe, an electrode, or another lesion-producing device. (The patient remains conscious throughout the procedure, permitting ongoing neurologic assessment.) When placed precisely, these lesions can cause analgesia. Stereotactic procedures can also be performed on the spinal cord.

CORDOTOMY

Surgical division of the spinothalamic tracts contralateral to the pain site by percutaneous radio frequency lesion or by direct visualization via laminectomy

Indications

Unilateral, below-the-waist pain from cancer; midline or bilateral pain (requires bilateral interruption of the spinothalamic tracts). Patient should have a life expectancy of less than 2 years.

Contraindications

Weakened or debilitated physical condition; inability to withstand the stress of surgery

Possible benefit

- Wide range of analgesia below the lesion

Risks

- Temporary sleep apnea (with high cervical bilateral percutaneous cordotomy)
- Bowel and bladder dysfunction (usually transient), sexual impotence, paralysis, and weakness (usually transient) in the arm and leg ipsilateral to the cordotomy

Note: Bilateral procedures are more likely to cause complications than unilateral procedures.

SYMPATHECTOMY

Surgical interruption of the sympathetic nerve pathways

Indications

Causalgia and pain associated with circulatory disorders, renal and urethral disorders, and biliary and pancreatic disease

Contraindication

Orthostatic hypotension

Possible benefits

- Eliminates vasospasms
- Dilates arterioles, increasing peripheral blood supply

Risks

- Ptosis
- Facial paralysis
- Masking of subsequent abdominal conditions
- Failure to relieve pain

Cordotomy

To perform this procedure, the doctor transects the lateral spinothalamic tract with a sharp, pointed blade. In this illustration, the shaded section indicates the transected area.

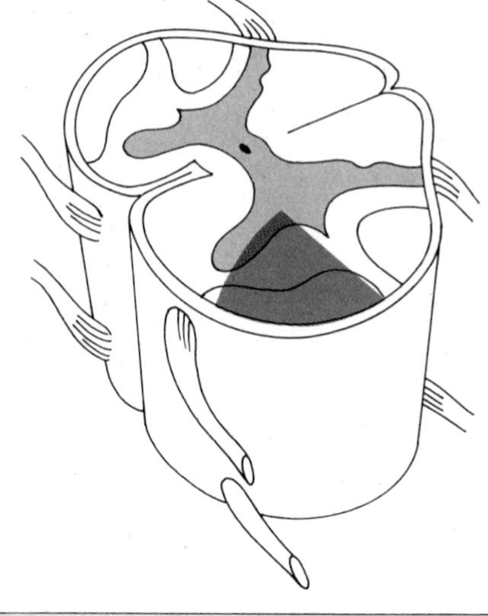

HYPOPHYSECTOMY

Surgical removal or chemical destruction of the pituitary gland

Indication

Bone pain from metastatic cancer

Contraindication

Pain not related to cancer

Possible benefits

- Reduction in tumor size
- Resolution of bone lesions

Risks

- Altered sex drive
- Impotence or infertility
- Hair loss
- Emotional lability

NEURECTOMY

Excision of a peripheral nerve

Indication

Pain well-localized within an area innervated by that peripheral nerve

Contraindication

Widespread pain

Possible benefit

- Relief of localized pain

Risks

- Failure to relieve pain
- Painful paresthesias

RHIZOTOMY

Surgical division of the nerve root as it enters the spinal cord; may be performed percutaneously or via laminectomy

Indications

Well-localized pain in the segmental distribution of a few sensory nerve roots from a localized malignant tumor, nerve entrapment from operative or traumatic scars, or herniated disks

Possible benefit

- Complete pain relief

Risks

- Complications associated with laminectomy
- Extremities may become useless if proprioception is not preserved and multiple roots are surgically divided
- Complete sensory loss
- Painful paresthesias

DORSAL ROOT ENTRY ZONE (DREZ) LESION

urgical destruction of Lissauer's ·act and the entry region of dorsal oot fibers in the spinal cord

ndication

ain secondary to brachial plexus vulsion

ossible benefit

Pain relief

isks

Cranial nerve damage

Recurrence of pain (rare)

TRACTOTOMY

nterruption of the spinothalamic ·act contralateral to the pain site t the medullary or mesencephalic evel

ndication

ain in the face, neck, and arm

ossible benefit

May produce analgesia at a higher egmental level than produced by ordotomy

isks

Decreased sensation in contralat- ·ral arm and side of face

Central dysesthesia

Recurrence of pain

CINGULOTOMY

)estruction of the medial white natter (cingulate bundle) with lectric current or ultrasound

ndications

)iffuse visceral or bone pain from netastatic cancer

ossible benefit

Modifies the patient's response to ain

isks

Recurrence of pain in several nonths, when surgery is unilateral

Personality changes (including rimitive asocial behavior, aggres- ion, or apathy), when surgery is ilateral

PREPARATION AND POSTOPERATIVE CARE

When your patient's scheduled for a neurosurgical procedure to relieve his pain, you're responsible for preparing him beforehand and caring for him afterward. Though most of your pre- and postoperative care is similar to what you'd give any surgical patient, the following points are particularly important.

Preoperative care

- After the doctor's explained the procedure, make sure the patient understands the expected benefits and possible risks associated with it. Clear up any misconceptions he has, and answer his questions.

If you can't answer all your patient's questions concerning the surgical procedure he's about to undergo, ask the doctor to speak with him again.

- Reassure the patient that postoperative pain (for example, incisional pain following a laminectomy) will be minimized. Also, prepare him for any unusual conditions that will result from the procedure. For example, if he's scheduled for a sympathectomy, inform him that the affected extremity won't perspire.
- Perform a baseline cranial nerve assessment and a neurologic check to permit meaningful postoperative evaluation.
- Make sure the doctor obtains written consent from the patient.

Postoperative care

- Check the patient's vital signs and level of consciousness every hour during the first 4 hours, every 4 hours for the next 48, and then once a shift (or as ordered).
- As ordered, change the dressings and apply antibiotic ointment to the incision every 24 hours or more frequently if the dressing becomes soiled or the site is exposed to air.
- Check the incision frequently for signs of bleeding, infection, cerebrospinal leakage, swelling, redness, or exudate. As ordered, give prophylactic antibiotics up to 7 days after the procedure.
- Regularly ask the patient if he's in pain or has any other distressing symptoms.
- Encourage him to engage in active range-of-motion exercises using his unaffected extremities. Help him perform passive range-of-motion exercises using his affected extremities.
- Perform frequent neurologic checks, including bilateral sensory and motor testing, cranial nerve checks, gait assessment (when the patient can get out of bed), and assessment of bowel and bladder function.
- Apply antiembolism stockings, if ordered.
- If your patient's had a hypophysectomy, elevate the head of the bed about 30° (as ordered) to promote venous drainage from his head and to reduce cerebral edema. To prevent cerebrospinal fluid drainage through nasal passages, don't permit your patient to blow his nose.
- If your patient's had a sympathectomy, observe him for signs and symptoms of neuritis, which may result from nerve manipulation during surgery. Tell him that this condition usually resolves spontaneously. Also monitor the patient for slight temperature increases in the lower extremities.

PAIN-CONTROL CENTERS

A FOCUSED APPROACH TO CHRONIC PAIN

Gone are the days when health-care professionals considered pain to be merely a symptom of some underlying disease or condition. Today, we recognize pain—particularly chronic pain—as a primary health-care problem equal to any other. In fact, pain is the leading reason people seek medical attention. According to the National Institutes of Health, pain is also the most expensive health problem—costing an estimated $50 billion a year. This, of course, doesn't begin to take into account its toll in human suffering.

As our awareness of pain as a distinct health-care problem has grown, so has our sophistication in dealing with it. In the early 1970s, Dr. John Bonica revolutionized thinking about chronic pain treatment by proposing a multidisciplinary approach to the problem. Today's pain-control centers (see Appendix) resulted from his efforts.

Clinic types. A pain-control center is a facility dedicated to the treatment and study of chronic pain. Perhaps because the concept is relatively new, centers differ widely in organization and emphasis. In general, however, they are multidisciplinary centers that draw on the talents of a variety of health-care professionals, including anesthesiologists, neurologists, neurosurgeons, psychiatrists, psychologists, pharmacists, dentists, and orthopedists. Patients can be treated as either inpatients or outpatients.

Goals. Although pain-control centers vary somewhat in their approach to treatment, they all share these goals:

- to diminish, if not eliminate, chronic pain
- to increase the patient's ability to function and lead a more active life
- to decrease the patient's dependence on drugs for pain control.

Patient teaching. If one of your patients is a long-term chronic pain sufferer, his doctor might refer him to a pain-control center for help. Chances are, the patient won't know what to expect. You can help prepare him by following these guidelines:

- Explain how the pain-control center is organized and what its goals are. Tell him that, although treatment programs vary among clinics, most involve group discussions and teaching sessions along with individual counseling.
- If he's currently taking pain medication, inform him that most clinics aim to gradually wean patients away from potent analgesics. But reassure him that medication withdrawal will progress gradually as he learns to function without medication or with only small doses of aspirin or another nonnarcotic analgesic.
- Prepare him for lengthy initial interviews by staff members. Tell him that these time-consuming interviews are designed to permit staff members to thoroughly evaluate his problem and devise a personalized care plan.
- Emphasize that referral to a pain-control center doesn't mean that you, the doctor, or other staff members think that his pain is imaginary. Make sure he understands that he'll be treated by health-care professionals who specialize in problems like his.

Who's running the pain-control centers?

A pain-control center's treatment approach is likely to reflect the director's area of expertise. As this illustration shows, anesthesiologists far outnumber directors from other disciplines. In a pain-control center headed by an anesthesiologist, the patient's initial treatment may include a diagnostic or therapeutic nerve block (see page 66).

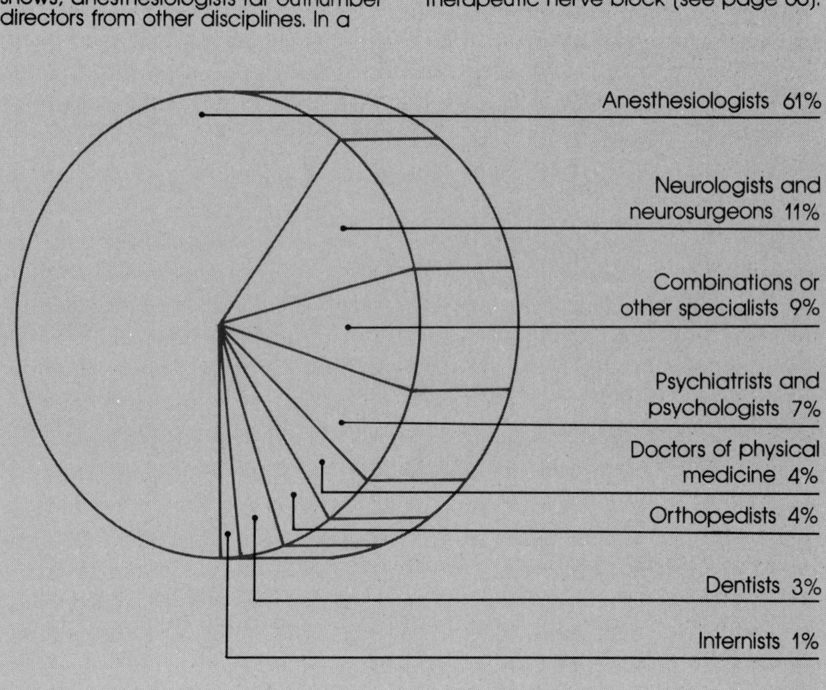

Source: Data compiled by the American Society of Anesthesiologists in the 1979 *Pain Clinic Directory.*

A SPECIAL PATIENT

Because pain-control centers attempt to help people with intractable pain, each patient presents a special challenge to the skills of every health team member. Consider, for example, the background of an average pain-center patient.

Patient profile. Typically, he's suffering chronic pain—lower back, headache, or phantom limb pain. He's probably endured pain for years, despite treatment by many doctors and therapists. By the time he arrives at the pain-control center, he may be financially drained, dependent on medication, anxious, depressed, and pessimistic after many discouraging years of unsuccessful treatment. In addition, he may bear the scars of numerous surgeries (on the average, pain-center patients have each undergone six surgeries). Because of his pain, he's probably coping with such problems as the inability to hold a job, mounting financial obligations, and strained personal relationships.

Not surprisingly, he spends many of his waking hours in bed. He exhibits frequent mood and affect changes that reflect his emotional condition as well as his physical dependence on prescription and nonprescription drugs.

As a result of his chronic pain, the patient withdraws from his family and friends and, in doing so, becomes socially isolated. He may have low self-esteem. A sense of hopelessness and helplessness sets in, and he becomes increasingly immobile. Possibly the most difficult characteristic to deal with is his dissatisfaction and even hostility toward all health-care professionals, including you.

Your role. If you're part of a pain center's multidisciplinary team, you play a pivotal role in teaching isolated, hopeless, and possibly distrustful patients. In either an inpatient or outpatient facility, you play an active role in assessing, planning, implementing, and evaluating pain and pain-management techniques.

Because the typical patient at a pain-control center has been through myriad unsuccessful pain treatments, he may be anxious about any new treatment. Knowing that one nurse is responsible for his care and treatment helps to reduce his anxiety.

Approximately one of every seven Americans has lower back pain at some time during his life: lower back pain partially disables five million people and severely disables two million more. Many never completely recover.

As a health team member, you must be ready to:

• establish a data base
• thoroughly assess the patient's pain
• formulate a nursing diagnosis
• work with the patient, his family, and other staff members to set long- and short-term goals
• conduct individual as well as group patient-teaching sessions
• instruct the patient in cognitive pain-relief techniques
• teach him how to use transcutaneous electrical nerve stimulation (TENS) to relieve pain, if required
• coordinate his medication and treatment schedule
• assist with such pain-control procedures as nerve blocks
• evaluate treatment and make adjustments, as necessary.

INVESTIGATING THE OPTIONS

Although all pain-control centers emphasize education, emotional support, physical conditioning, and cognitive strategies, their specific approaches to treatment vary. Some centers (for example, nerve block clinics) emphasize one particular pain treatment; others are multidisciplinary.

Centers can offer inpatient programs, outpatient programs, or both. Here's how inpatient and outpatient programs compare.

Inpatient programs. Based on such strategies as behavior modification, stress management, relaxation training, and other cognitive therapies, inpatient programs prepare the patient to function in spite of his pain. Most programs also offer physical therapy, occupational therapy, patient and family teaching, and drug detoxification programs.

Centers offering inpatient programs vary in size and expense (from $8,000 to $24,000 for an average 4- to 6-week stay). Two major advantages of this type of program include:

• round-the-clock monitoring (necessary for most drug detoxification programs)
• a consistent, structured environment that supports rehabilitation.

Outpatient programs. While regularly attending prescribed outpatient classes, the patient learns to integrate new pain-control strategies into his everyday life. Although most outpatient centers don't offer the extensive psychological conditioning programs of their inpatient counterparts, they offer many of the same services, such as physical and occupational therapy, patient and family teaching, and drug detoxification programs. In addition to being less expensive, outpatient programs allow the patient to continue his usual life-style.

PAIN-CONTROL CENTERS CONTINUED

ONE PATIENT'S HISTORY

Two years ago, Lorraine Angle, a 35-year-old nurse and divorced mother of two teenagers, injured her back while lifting a patient. Her doctor suspected a herniated disk and admitted her to the hospital for conservative treatment. After her condition improved, she was discharged.

During the next year, Mrs. Angle was admitted to the hospital three times for bed rest and physical therapy. Because conservative measures hadn't relieved her pain, the doctor ordered a myelogram, which confirmed the presence of a herniated lumbar disk. He then performed a lumbar laminectomy.

After a 3-week hospital stay, she was discharged. Although her back pain hadn't been eliminated, it was under control. As soon as her doctor gave his approval, she returned to work.

Two days later, she was involved in an automobile accident. The jolt caused her lower back pain to flare up again—worse than before. With the support of a back brace she could walk, but the pain made returning to work impossible.

To control her pain, the doctor prescribed these drugs, p.r.n.: the skeletal muscle relaxant Robaxisal, oxycodone hydrochloride (Percodan), and lorazepam (Ativan). Unfortunately, these drugs brought only partial relief.

Meanwhile, she continued to have setbacks. Occasional falls exacerbated her pain. Unable to work, she became increasingly anxious about her dwindling financial resources. To help Mrs. Angle find ways to cope with her problems, the doctor referred her to a pain-control center. To find out how a patient like Mrs. Angle might be treated, read what follows.

TREATING MRS. ANGLE: TWO APPROACHES

What kind of treatment can Mrs. Angle expect at the pain-control center? That depends on whether she's treated as an inpatient or an outpatient. Here are two possible approaches and how you would fit in with each one.

Inpatient. Your first responsibility during Mrs. Angle's 4-week stay is to perform a complete pain assessment. Help develop an individualized treatment approach based on your findings and the evaluations of other health-care members. Goals for Mrs. Angle's stay are to:

- decrease pain
- improve self-esteem
- reduce reliance on narcotics
- return to work
- increase function
- strengthen coping skills.

To achieve these goals, Mrs. Angle participates in several highly structured daily activities: relaxation class, walking, group therapy (to discuss stress management, life-style changes, discharge planning, relaxation techniques, and assertiveness training), physical and occupational therapy, keeping a pain and mood record, swimming, and attending a class on natural pain-control techniques.

To reduce her dependence on narcotics, the health team uses this approach: Mrs. Angle takes her medications on a fixed schedule. All medications are provided in liquid or capsule form, and all look alike—preventing her from knowing which drugs she's taking. As ordered, the health team gradually reduces drug doses.

At the end of 1 week, the health team evaluates Mrs. Angle's progress toward controlling her pain, her drug schedule, and her emotional condition. Because she's responding well, the health team continues with this approach for the remaining 3 weeks of her stay.

Outpatient. Now suppose that Mrs. Angle entered the center as an outpatient. Your first responsibility is to take a history and to thoroughly assess her pain. Teach her to keep a pain diary, and arrange for evaluations by the center's doctor, psychologist, and physical therapist.

After the initial evaluations, the multidisciplinary health team meets and sets these goals:

- to break the pain cycle by administering myoneural blocks into the lower back every 2 weeks for 6 weeks
- to reduce analgesics over several months
- to increase the strength of abdominal muscles and back extensors, increase flexibility in the lower back, increase leg strength, increase endurance and tolerance to movement, and help reverse tissue atrophy from muscle guarding with exercise under the supervision of a physical therapist
- to reduce pain with biofeedback, relaxation, and self-hypnosis.

During Mrs. Angle's next visit to the pain center, you discuss her goals and coordinate a schedule that meets her needs: nerve-block treatment, physical therapy, cognitive behavioral therapy, and education classes on such topics as sleep, nutrition, medication, stress management, and relaxation.

Outcome. Whether you helped to treat Mrs. Angle on an inpatient or an outpatient basis, you aimed for the same results. After successful treatment, she can resume a normal life-style. Her pain is under control. No longer dependent on narcotics, she takes only small doses of acetaminophen. In short, Mrs. Angle has regained a sense of well-being and feels in control of her life.

DRUG THERAPY

- PHARMACOKINETICS
- ANALGESIA
- N.S.A.I.D.s
- NARCOTICS
- MORPHINE
- ADJUVANT DRUGS
- LACEBOS
- ANALGESIC GUIDELINES
- SPECIAL INFUSION SYSTEMS

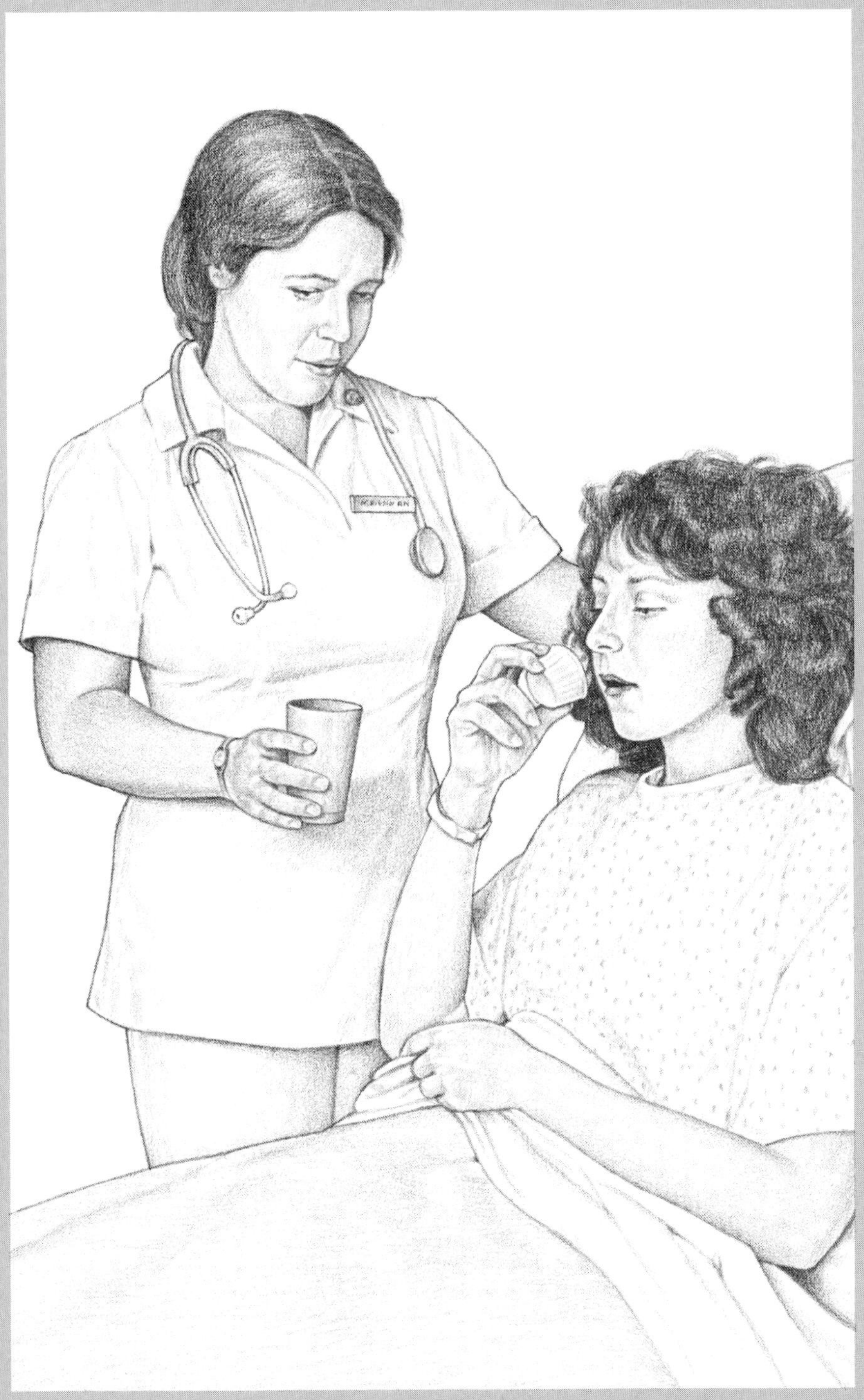

PHARMACOKINETICS

WHAT INFLUENCES DRUG PROCESSING?

Why is an oral analgesic such as codeine highly effective for one patient yet ineffective for another patient with similar pain? To answer this question, you need to know how *pharmacokinetics* (drug processing in the body) affects *pharmacodynamics* (patient response).

Pharmacokinetics encompasses four basic processes that occur when a drug enters the body: absorption, distribution, metabolism, and excretion. Any factor that affects one or more of these processes also affects your patient's response to the drug. Among the many influences on drug processing and patient response are the following:

- drug composition, which determines where and how the drug is absorbed, the areas it's distributed to, where (at what sites) it's metabolized, and how quickly it's excreted
- the patient's condition and its effect on liver and kidney function
- the administration route
- the amount of drug administered
- the drug's potential to interact with other drugs the patient is taking
- the patient's potential to develop a tolerance to the drug.

When you understand what happens to drugs as they pass through the body, you'll be prepared to take action *before* problems arise. For example, you'll know that the oral form of a drug may not be the best choice for a patient with severe diarrhea—because the drug may not remain in his gastrointestinal tract long enough for absorption to occur. And when a problem with a drug does arise, you'll understand why and be ready to take immediate corrective measures. For details on each phase of drug processing—from absorption to excretion—read the next few pages.

ABSORPTION: THE FIRST STEP

Absorption occurs when a drug is transported into the patient's circulatory system from the point where it was administered. How quickly and completely a drug is absorbed influences its onset, duration, and intensity of action.

Administration route. Drug route influences the amount and the rate of absorption. When you give a drug I.V., its absorption is immediate and complete—the drug is 100% bioavailable. But a drug given by any other route has to penetrate one or more lipid cell-membrane barriers before it reaches the circulatory system. *Note:* With intramuscular and subcutaneous injections, blood supply at the injection site is an important factor affecting absorption.

For orally administered drugs, the process is more complex. An oral drug given in tablet or capsule form must dissolve in the GI tract before absorption can occur.

Factors affecting GI absorption. A number of factors can affect a drug's absorption in the GI tract. This can make oral drug dosage difficult to determine.

When an oral drug enters the GI tract, its absorption is affected by stomach emptying time, changing pH in the GI tract, the presence (or absence) of food, and GI motility.

What about your patient's condition? A few factors diminish drug absorption in the GI tract:

- bowel resection or obstruction
- vomiting and diarrhea
- low stomach acid content
- the presence of other drugs or food, which may bind the drug and prevent absorption.

Intestinal villi

Each intestinal villus contains a network of veins, arteries, and lymph channels, as shown here in the cross section. The microvilli covering each villus further increase intestinal surface area, promoting absorption.

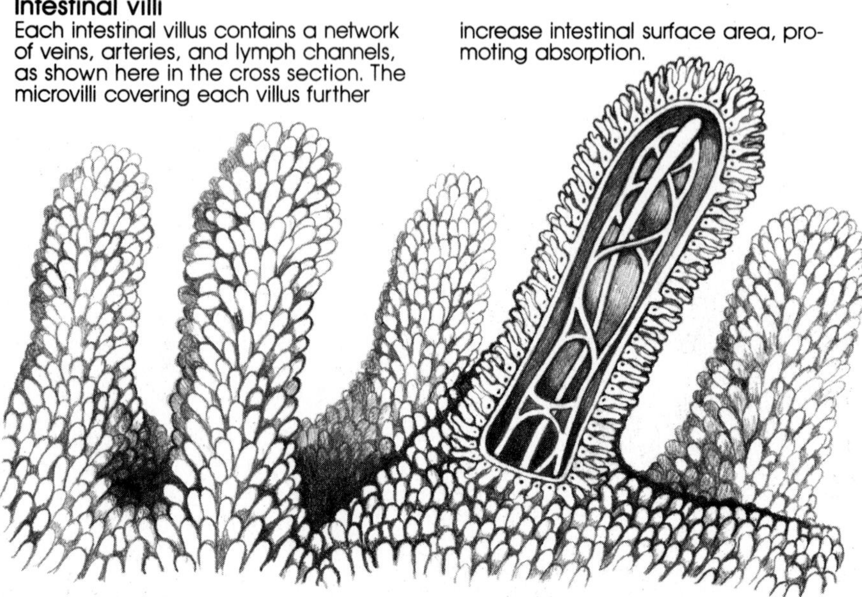

DISTRIBUTION: THE SECOND STEP

Once a drug is absorbed, it's distributed throughout your patient's system. For most drugs, the intended therapeutic effect (or unintended adverse effect) takes place during the distribution phase.

As drug molecules are absorbed into the bloodstream, some bind to plasma proteins or red blood cells while others remain free. Both bound and free molecules are carried by the bloodstream to the body's fluid compartments and tissues.

Because drug distribution takes place via the bloodstream, a patient's circulatory status affects delivery of drug molecules to tissues. Drug molecules are quick to reach highly vascular organs and slow to reach less vascular tissue, such as muscle, fat, and skin. (Although the brain is highly vascular, the blood-brain barrier blocks distribution of many drugs to this organ.)

After distribution to tissue, free drug molecules combine with *receptors*—parts of the cell membrane that interact with drugs to produce a therapeutic effect. Most receptors are proteins or nucleic acids, though enzymes, lipids, and carbohydrate residues can also act as receptors. For a drug to be effective, its molecules must bind with receptors that have the right chemical fit. Since receptors combine normally with naturally produced chemicals to regulate body processes, most drugs mimic or block the action of the natural chemical.

Only free drug molecules combine with receptors—but bound drug molecules also play a role. When released gradually, bound drug molecules can keep the bound/unbound ratio constant, contributing to a predictable, uniform therapeutic effect.

METABOLISM: PREPARING FOR EXCRETION

Metabolism (also called biotransformation) is an interaction between a drug (or other substance) and an enzyme. The enzyme remains unchanged by the interaction, but the drug is broken down into *metabolites.* Although most metabolism takes place in the liver, some metabolism also occurs in the intestinal walls, plasma, and kidneys.

Metabolism usually changes lipid-soluble drug molecules into a more water-soluble form. For *inbound* passage, the more lipid-soluble a drug is, the easier it crosses cell membranes for absorption and distribution. But water solubility makes the drug easier to excrete.

Active or inactive. Because of the different biochemical reactions taking place during drug metabolism, some metabolites are pharmacologically *inactive* whereas others are pharmacologically *active.* Some drugs (called *prodrugs*) are inactive when they're administered and don't become active until they're transformed into metabolites. A few drugs—such as codeine and its metabolite morphine—are active in *both* their administered and metabolized forms.

Note: Active metabolites can produce both therapeutic and toxic effects. For example, meperidine's metabolite normeperidine is potentially neurotoxic. When given in high repetitive doses, it may cause convulsions in patients with renal dysfunction.

Metabolic rate. Just as absorption rate affects a drug's effectiveness, the rate of drug metabolism influences the duration and the intensity of the drug's action. Each patient has a different rate of drug metabolism, which is influenced by age, disease (especially of the liver), the presence of other drugs in the system, and genetic factors that alter the presence or efficiency of enzymes involved in drug metabolism.

You can see, then, why a drug may be metabolized quickly in one patient yet build to toxic levels in another patient.

How first-pass metabolism affects oral drugs

You've probably given many parenteral doses of meperidine (Demerol) but few (if any) oral doses. And if you've given meperidine in oral form, you were probably surprised to see how much larger the oral dose was.

The reason is *first-pass metabolism,* a process that occurs when the portal vein brings blood containing nutrients and orally administered drugs from the GI tract directly to the liver. A considerable percentage of these drugs may be metabolized in the liver and sent to the kidneys for excretion before they ever reach the intended receptor sites.

Oral doses of drugs cleared by first-pass metabolism must be given in larger doses to ensure a therapeutic effect. Meperidine is one such drug.

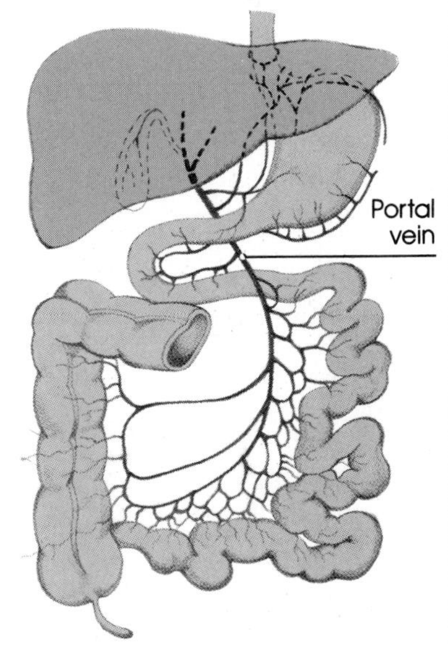

PHARMACOKINETICS CONTINUED

EXCRETION: THE FINAL PHASE

Most drugs are primarily excreted in urine via the kidneys; some, however, are excreted via the lungs or in feces, saliva, sweat, breast milk (in lactating women), or bile, which can carry metabolized drug to the small intestine for excretion or reabsorption.

If drug excretion is delayed, the drug remains in the patient's system longer—and the drug's effects are long-lasting. Because most drugs are excreted primarily by the kidneys, any disease or condition that compromises kidney function also delays drug excretion. Other causes of delayed excretion include drug interactions and impaired cardiovascular or liver function.

For most drugs, the duration of action correlates roughly with the drug's *half-life*—the time it takes for half of the drug to be eliminated from the body. Methadone, however, is one of many exceptions to this rule. Although its half-life is 17 to 24 hours, you may need to give it every 3 to 4 hours to maintain analgesia.

Standard dosage intervals are based on the drug's half-life (or, for drugs such as methadone, its duration of effect). These figures are helpful in setting up a dosage schedule that builds to a plateau or *steady state*—the state of equilibrium in which the amount of drug leaving the system equals the amount of drug administered. In general, a steady state occurs after approximately four half-lives. Dosage intervals are calculated to maintain steady state concentration below the toxic level but above the minimum therapeutic level.

Achieving a steady state

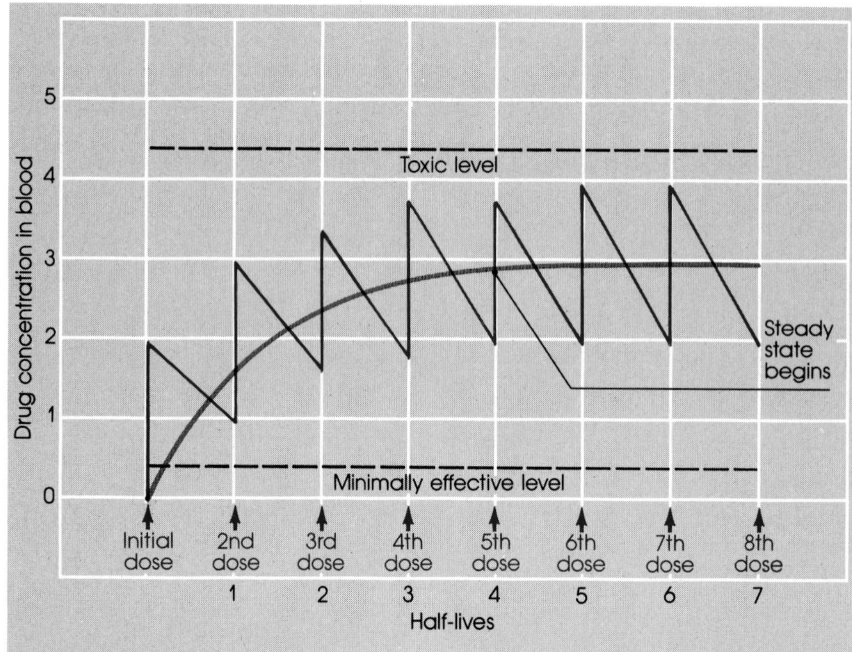

To establish a steady state of drug concentration in the blood, the doctor orders dosages based on the drug's half-life or duration of effect. As shown above, drug levels reach a steady state after four or five doses. (A steady state is achieved faster when therapy begins with a loading dose.)

ANALGESIA

ANALGESICS AND THE PATIENT IN PAIN: BALANCING THE EFFECTS

An analgesic isn't the only way to relieve a patient's pain. But because it modifies your patient's perception of pain (without causing a loss of consciousness), it's considered one of the most reliable, effective, and fast-acting methods of pain relief available for various conditions.

An analgesic's effect on your patient's pain depends on several factors: the pain's severity, the drug chosen, the dosage, the route, the time of administration, and the patient's individual response to the drug. For all of these reasons, an analgesic that works well for one patient in pain may produce adverse effects in another patient with a similar painful condition.

What can you do to ensure optimum pain relief from an analgesic? First, you can learn more about the three main analgesic categories: nonsteroidal anti-inflammatory drugs (NSAIDs), narcotics, and adjuvants. This will help familiarize you with the analgesic options available to your patient. Then you can learn how to achieve an effective balance between an analgesic's pain-relieving properties and its adverse effects. Begin with the following review.

NSAIDs. Nonsteroidal anti-inflammatory drugs is an umbrella term covering a large group of compounds that modify the inflammatory response by interfering with the synthesis of prostaglandins, which appear to sensitize pain receptors. By reducing local heat, swelling, and stiffness, these drugs control pain at the peripheral nervous system level. They also act centrally, although no one is sure how. Prime examples of NSAIDs include acetylsalicylic acid (aspirin), acetaminophen (Tylenol), and ibuprofen (Motrin).

Note: Although acetaminophen is classified as an NSAID, its anti-inflammatory action is clinically insignificant.

Narcotics. To alter the perception of pain and emotional response to it, narcotics bind with opiate receptors in the central nervous system. Unlike NSAIDs, these drugs may cause tolerance or physical dependence with long-term use. They're usually given to patients with severe acute pain and chronic pain associated with cancer.

Narcotic analgesics act centrally to induce analgesia; they also depress respirations and cause nausea, vomiting, and constipation.

Commonly ordered narcotics include: morphine, meperidine hydrochloride (Demerol), and propoxyphene hydrochloride (Darvon*).

Adjuvants. These central-acting drugs are given mainly with narcotics to potentiate the beneficial effects of narcotics and to counteract their adverse effects. Examples of adjuvants are such anticonvulsants as phenytoin (Dilantin) and carbamazepine (Tegretol), and such antihistamines as hydroxyzine (Vistaril*).

*Not available in Canada

ANALGESIC USE AND ABUSE: DOES YOUR PATIENT KNOW BEST?

"Can you give me something for my pain?" asks the patient in room 214C.

Not surprisingly, many patients say they fear pain more than anything else during hospitalization. And yet, many nurses and other health-care professionals hesitate to provide adequate pain-relief medication for fear of over-medicating patients and, in turn, nurturing drug dependence. As a result, some patients suffer needlessly.

You can avoid being misled by the myths associated with analgesic use by knowing the facts.

• *Myth 1: Analgesics don't relieve pain when anxiety is a strong component.* Remember, pain and anxiety reinforce each other. The central nervous system activity that accompanies pain heightens anxiety; as anxiety grows, pain intensifies. By relieving pain, analgesics can also reduce pain-related anxiety.

Remember, pain is what your patient says it is. Take all pain complaints seriously, and intervene appropriately.

• *Myth 2: A patient who asks for pain medication at regular intervals or in increasing amounts is a potential addict.* In all probability, a patient demanding pain medication every 2 to 3 hours (or in increasing amounts) is a patient with poorly controlled pain—not a potential addict.

Fear of drug addiction or dependence is a major concern of patients, families, and health-care professionals alike. Rarely, though, does a medical patient without a history of drug addiction become psychologically dependent on drugs. (According to one study, less than 1% of hospitalized patients receiving narcotic analgesics become psychologically addicted.)

Take care not to label a patient who's physically dependent on medication an addict. Physical dependence is an expected effect after 2 or more weeks of narcotic use. Labeling a patient only interferes with your ability to provide quality care.

• *Myth 3: To prevent abuse, give analgesics only on demand.* Although an *as needed* (p.r.n.) medication schedule is appropriate in some cases, it can be woefully inadequate for severe acute pain and for some types of chronic pain. Why? Because by the time the patient requests medication, he already may be experiencing severe pain. And, as you know, one key to controlling pain is to treat it as soon as it begins, before it gets out of hand.

When such a patient isn't medicated regularly—before pain begins—a vicious cycle may result: as the patient anticipates the onset of severe pain, his anxiety increases and his pain worsens. If administered regularly, however, pain medication can decrease the patient's anxiety, in turn reducing his pain.

• *Myth 4: The most effective way to give narcotics is by injection.* Unless you're familiar with oral/parenteral ratios, this may seem true. But with appropriate dosage adjustments, many narcotics work well in oral form and provide the patient with the same pain relief he'd obtain from parenteral administration. In addition, oral narcotic use is associated with slower development of tolerance than parenteral use; it's also more convenient and less painful.

ANALGESIA CONTINUED

KNOWING YOUR RESPONSIBILITIES

You're right if you think administering analgesics is a big responsibility. Although doctors order analgesics, they rely on you to administer the medication properly, evaluate its effectiveness, watch for side effects, and inform them of the patient's progress. In many cases, your nursing judgment makes the difference between successful or unsuccessful pain-relief therapy. After all, you spend more time with your patient than any other health-care professional does, so you're in a better position to determine how well he responds to a specific analgesic.

To administer an analgesic properly you first have to accept responsibility for interpreting the doctor's order and administering the drug correctly. Don't take the easy way out by throwing the burden of responsibility on the doctor ("This order should be more specific"), the patient ("He should remember what he was taking for his pain"), or the drug ("Why doesn't the package insert tell you how effective it is?"). Your knowledge of the patient and the analgesic you're administering is essential. Assume the following responsibilities—and consider yourself liable for them.

- Make sure you're well informed about all the drugs you administer. In addition to knowing indications, contraindications, expected effects, and possible adverse effects, take note of the onset of action and peak effect periods for each drug. All this information helps you to identify adverse reactions if they occur and to intervene appropriately. If your patient suffers an adverse reaction, note his signs and symptoms, when they occurred, and what drugs he received before the reaction.
- When the doctor orders a drug given p.r.n., regularly assess the patient for pain, administer medication as needed, and take responsibility for pain management.
- When the doctor prescribes more than one drug for pain relief, determine which one is indicated. (We'll discuss how to make this judgment in the following pages.)
- Determine analgesic effectiveness through ongoing patient assessment. The data you obtain helps you and the doctor know how well your intervention is relieving the patient's pain.
- Inform the doctor immediately when analgesic changes are needed. Be prepared to give specific reasons, and offer a few suggestions. Based on your patient assessment, you may recommend increasing or decreasing the dosage, switching to another analgesic, adding another analgesic, or reducing the time between doses.
- Teach the patient and his family about the use of prescription and over-the-counter analgesics. Dispel myths they may have heard, and teach them how to use analgesics safely and effectively. Answer any questions they have, and refer them to the pharmacist or doctor for questions you can't answer.

N.S.A.I.D.s

KEY CONCEPTS

Although you're well acquainted with such drugs as aspirin, acetaminophen, and ibuprofen, you may be less familiar with the umbrella term that covers them: nonsteroidal anti-inflammatory drugs (NSAIDs). You may be accustomed to calling them *nonnarcotic analgesics.*

NSAIDs encompass a group of structurally different nonsteroidal drugs that produce similar effects in the body. Although they work by different mechanisms, all NSAIDs have anti-inflammatory, antipyretic, and analgesic properties. However, these properties vary widely from drug to drug. Acetaminophen, for example, has only minor anti-inflammatory effects; aspirin has major anti-inflammatory effects.

Although mechanisms of action are complex and not completely understood, the antipyretic effects of NSAIDs are believed to be mediated centrally at the hypothalamus, the body's temperature regulation center.

Anti-inflammatory and analgesic effects are apparently produced both centrally and peripherally. How NSAIDs produce these effects at the central level isn't well understood. But at the peripheral level, these drugs act by modifying the inflammatory cascade.

The doctor orders NSAIDs to relieve mild-to-moderate pain. In combination with narcotic analgesics, they're also effective against moderate-to-severe pain.

Because NSAIDs vary in chemical structure, their onset of action, duration of effect, metabolism, and elimination differ. In addition, what works for one patient's pain may be ineffective against another patient's pain. The doctor may try several drugs before finding one that's effective for your patient.

SOME EXAMPLES

The following drugs are classified as NSAIDs:

- acetaminophen (Tylenol)
- aspirin (A.S.A.*)
- fenoprofen calcium (Nalfon)
- ibuprofen (Advil*, Motrin, Nuprin*)
- indomethacin (Indocin*)
- meclofenamate (Meclomen*)
- mefenamic acid (Ponstel*)
- naproxen (Naprosyn)
- naproxen sodium (Anaprox*)
- oxyphenbutazone (Tandearil*)
- phenylbutazone (Butazolidin)
- piroxicam (Feldene*)
- sulindac (Clinoril*)
- tolmetin sodium (Tolectin)

BLOCKING PAIN AT THE PERIPHERAL LEVEL

As you learned on page 12, prostaglandins sensitize pain receptors and stimulate pain-impulse transmission. When acting at the peripheral level, most NSAIDs apparently interrupt prostaglandin synthesis, as shown in the illustration at right.

After injury, cells release histamine and bradykinin precursors, and arachidonic acid is formed. Normally, an enzyme called prostaglandin synthetase (cyclo-oxygenase enzyme complex) acts on arachidonic acid, leading to prostaglandin synthesis. NSAIDs, in their role as prostaglandin inhibitors, inhibit prostaglandin synthetase and prevent prostaglandin formation.

Note: Aspirin irreversibly blocks prostaglandin synthetase; other NSAIDs are reversible inhibitors.

*Not available in Canada

How NSAIDs interrupt the inflammatory process

NSAIDs inhibit the inflammatory process, but they don't halt it. Other aspects of the inflammatory process, such as release of histamine and bradykinin precursors, continue unchecked.

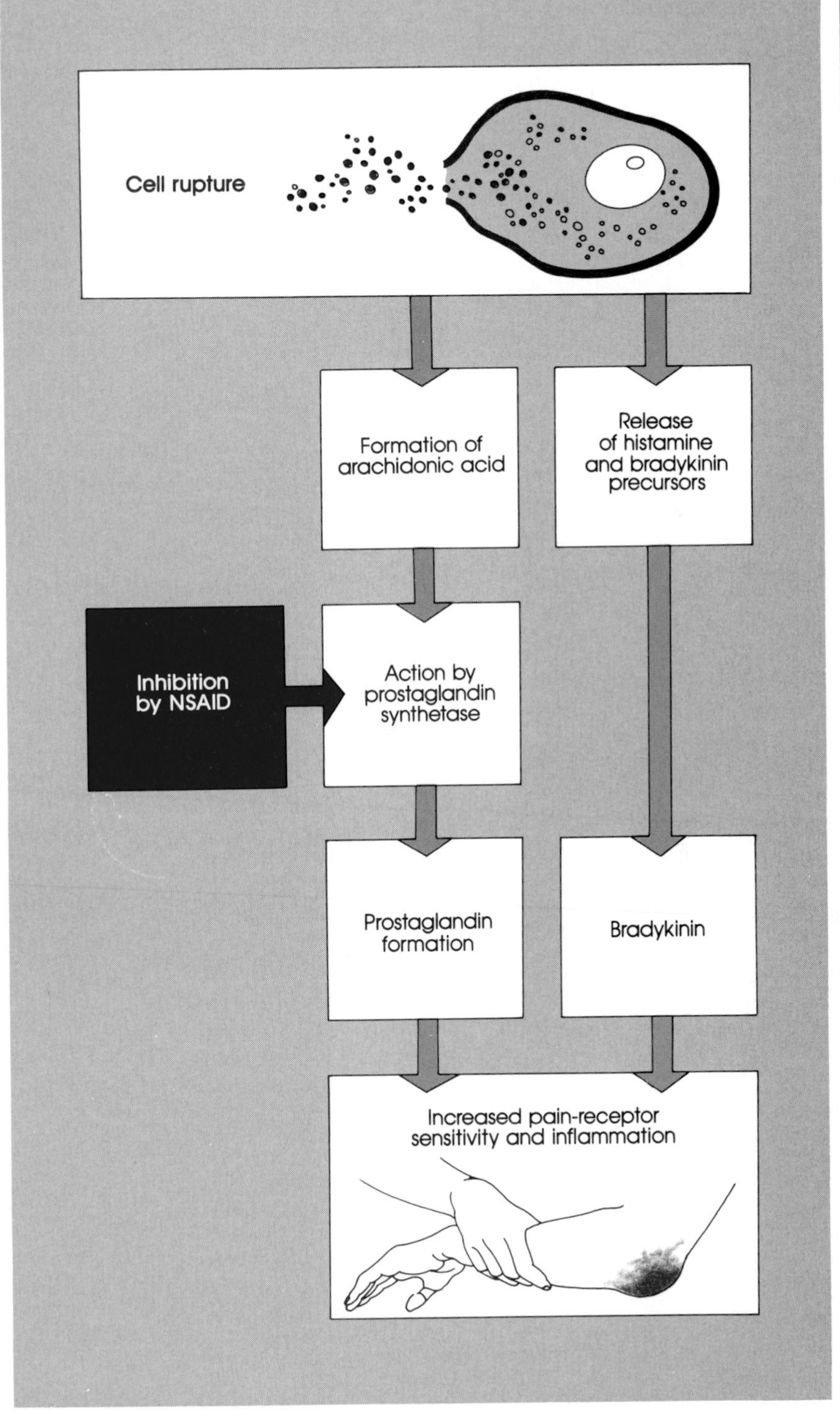

N.S.A.I.D.s CONTINUED

INDICATIONS FOR USE

NSAIDs are most effective for mild-to-moderate pain—especially pain associated with inflammation. Conditions for which they're commonly ordered include:

- migraine headache
- dysmenorrhea
- rheumatoid arthritis
- ankylosing spondylitis
- osteoarthritis
- gout
- bone pain, especially associated with metastatic disease.

"You've heard about them—the new aspirin products that seem to appear every week, promising faster disintegration, faster dissolution, less GI upset. The fact is, none of these new products has yet proven to be safer or more effective than the simple aspirin tablet.

If a patient can't take aspirin because he has a history of GI problems, he probably won't be able to take any of these fancy aspirin products either. Encourage him to substitute acetaminophen or (at his doctor's direction) another NSAID such as ibuprofen."

Larry Neil Gever, RPh, PharmD
Springhouse, Pa.

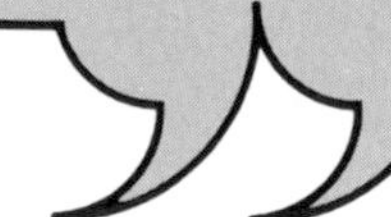

HOW THREE O.T.C. DRUGS COMPARE

These three commonly ordered NSAIDs—aspirin, acetaminophen, and ibuprofen—are available over the counter. But although all three drugs have analgesic effects, one may be better suited to your patient's condition than the others. The following chart details advantages and disadvantages you should teach your patient.

ASPIRIN
A.S.A.*, Ecotrin

Advantages

- Has a clinically significant anti-inflammatory effect
- Is inexpensive

Disadvantages

- Is contraindicated for patients prone to GI bleeding and for patients with low platelet counts
- May lead to *salicylism* (toxic effects characterized by tinnitus, nausea, and vomiting) if daily doses exceed 4 g
- May cause adverse effects to outweigh benefits with long-term use
- Is implicated in many adverse drug interactions
- Increases the risk of hypersensitivity reaction, especially in asthma patients
- Isn't available in liquid form

ACETAMINOPHEN
Tylenol

Advantages

- May be given to patients with low platelet counts and patients prone to GI bleeding
- May be given to patients who are hypersensitive to aspirin
- Has less potential for drug interactions than aspirin. However, taking acetaminophen for longer than 2 weeks may increase the risk of bleeding in patients taking oral anticoagulants.
- Enhances analgesia with doses greater than 650 mg
- Is inexpensive
- Is available in liquid form

Disadvantages

- May alter liver function tests and cause liver toxicity after prolonged use with doses greater than 4 g daily
- Has no clinically significant anti-inflammatory effect

IBUPROFEN
Advil*, Motrin, Nuprin*

Advantages

- May be effective for patients who don't respond to aspirin or acetaminophen
- Causes fewer adverse effects with long-term use than does aspirin. Ibuprofen is less irritating to GI mucosa and is less likely to cause bleeding.
- Has a clinically significant anti-inflammatory effect

Disadvantages

- Is more expensive than aspirin and acetaminophen
- Must be administered with caution in patients with a history of GI bleeding
- May lead to diminished renal function or nephrotoxicity with long-term use
- Is contraindicated for patients hypersensitive to aspirin
- Isn't available in liquid form
- May cause sodium and water retention

*Not available in Canada

ORAL N.S.A.I.D.S COMMONLY USED FOR MILD-TO-MODERATE PAIN

Drug	Usual dosage	Onset of analgesic action	Duration of analgesic action	Half-life
acetaminophen	325 to 975 mg q 4 hours p.r.n.	0.5 hour	4 hours	1.25 to 3 hours
aspirin	325 to 650 mg* q 4 hours p.r.n.	0.5 hour	4 hours	15 to 20 minutes
diflunisal	500 mg twice daily	1 hour	8 to 12 hours	8 to 12 hours
fenoprofen	200 mg q 4 to 6 hours p.r.n.	0.5 to 1 hour	4 to 6 hours	2 to 3 hours
ibuprofen	200 to 400 mg q 4 to 6 hours p.r.n.	0.5 hours	4 to 6 hours	1.8 to 2.5 hours
mefenamic acid	500 mg initially, then 250 mg q 6 hours p.r.n.	1 hour	6 hours	2 to 4 hours
naproxen	500 mg initially, then 250 mg q 6 to 8 hours p.r.n.	1 hour	up to 7 hours	12 to 15 hours
naproxen sodium	550 mg initially, then 275 mg q 6 to 8 hours p.r.n.	1 hour	up to 7 hours	12 to 15 hours

*Some patients may need up to 975 mg for analgesia.

ADVERSE EFFECTS: WHAT TO WATCH FOR

For most patients, NSAIDs are safe as well as effective. But like all drugs, they carry a risk of adverse effects. Here's what you should know.

GI irritation. The ability of NSAIDs to inhibit prostaglandin synthesis—a key to the drugs' anti-inflammatory and analgesic properties—also explains why dyspepsia, gastric irritation, and GI bleeding are adverse effects. As you know, prostaglandins are found throughout the body and fulfill a variety of functions in addition to mediating the inflammatory response. In the GI tract, prostaglandins increase mucous formation and decrease gastric acid production. By blocking prostaglandin synthesis in the GI tract, NSAIDs permit increased gastric acid production and decreased mucous formation. Both effects set the stage for GI irritation. (Uncoated aspirin is more likely to cause GI irritation than other NSAIDs.) NSAIDs also increase the risk of GI bleeding because of their effect on platelets, as we'll discuss next.

Monitor your patient for GI distress or discomfort. To minimize GI irritation, suggest that he take the drug with food, unless contraindicated. Use extreme caution if the patient has a history of GI problems, especially ulcers.

Bleeding. In addition to local GI effects, NSAIDs systemically prolong bleeding time by interfering with the prostaglandin-mediated clotting cascade.

Normally, the prostaglandin synthetase in platelets contributes to their ability to aggregate. Because aspirin irreversibly blocks prostaglandin synthetase, it has a greater effect on clotting time than other NSAIDs. In fact, a single 650-mg dose of aspirin approximately doubles bleeding time for 4 to 7 days. For this reason, aspirin is contraindicated for at least 1 week before surgery. (Other NSAIDs may be

CONTINUED ON PAGE 82

N.S.A.I.D.s CONTINUED

ADVERSE EFFECTS: WHAT TO WATCH FOR CONTINUED

given up to 1 day before surgery, as ordered.) Aspirin is also contraindicated for patients with hemophilia, severe liver disease or damage, hypothrombinemia, and vitamin K deficiency.

Blood dyscrasias. Prolonged use of oxyphenbutazone and phenylbutazone may increase the risk of aplastic anemia or agranulocytosis—both potentially fatal.

Hypersensitivity. A patient who's allergic or sensitive to aspirin may also be sensitive to other NSAIDs (except for acetaminophen, which has an extremely low potential for aspirin cross-sensitivity). Always inquire about aspirin sensitivity before giving any NSAID. In addition, use special caution if your patient has asthma. Aspirin can trigger *aspirin-induced asthma* (bronchoconstriction and possibly anaphylaxis) in some patients.

Sodium and water retention. When NSAIDs inhibit prostaglandin synthesis, they also alter the regulatory role of prostaglandins in renal blood flow. The result is sodium and water retention. Water retention can cause congestive heart failure and worsen preexisting hypertension.

Analgesic nephropathy. Recent studies show that nephropathy also may be linked to the long-term use of combination analgesics, including NSAIDs. Analgesic nephropathy is characterized by papillary necrosis and chronic interstitial nephritis.

Other effects. Long-term use of NSAIDs may cause interstitial nephritis and hepatotoxicity. Unpredictable and idiosyncratic, these effects can usually be reversed by discontinuing the drug.

To help avert interstitial nephritis, closely monitor renal function and alert the doctor to any change, especially in elderly patients and in those taking diuretics. Other patients at risk include those with diabetes mellitus, dehydration, preexisting renal dysfunction, congestive heart failure, and ascites.

Hepatotoxicity is most common in children and in patients with systemic lupus erythematosus. Acetaminophen poses a particular risk for hepatotoxicity.

Observe for increases in serum transaminase levels, and monitor liver function tests. With continued use, intracanalicular bile plugs and irreversible liver cell damage are possible.

INTERACTIONS: WHICH DRUGS DON'T MIX?

Your patient probably will be receiving drugs in addition to NSAIDs, putting him at risk of adverse effects from drug interactions. Depending on the drugs he's taking, he could also receive diminished therapeutic benefits from one or more drugs, unless dosage is adjusted appropriately.

Drug interactions. Read what follows for details you should know.

- Other anti-inflammatory medications (such as corticosteroids), taken concurrently with NSAIDs, increase the risk of adverse GI effects and ulcers. Closely monitor the patient for GI problems.
- Anticoagulants (such as warfarin sodium [Coumadin] or heparin) may be potentiated by aspirin, fenoprofen, meclofenamate, mefenamic acid, or sulindac. When giving NSAIDs and anticoagulants concurrently, monitor coagulation studies and adjust the anticoagulant dosage as ordered. NSAIDs, which inhibit platelet function, also increase the risk of GI ulceration or hemorrhage when given with anticoagulants.
- Naproxen and indomethacin may decrease the antihypertensive effect of furosemide (Lasix). As ordered, increase the dosage of furosemide.
- Indomethacin may increase serum lithium levels, risking toxicity. As ordered, decrease the dosage of lithium when giving it with indomethacin. Closely monitor serum lithium levels and patient response to therapy.
- Indomethacin decreases beta blockers' antihypertensive effect. Increase the dosage of beta blockers, as ordered, when giving them with indomethacin. Closely monitor the patient's blood pressure during therapy.

Other interactions. Besides interacting with other drugs, NSAIDs can induce physiologic changes that alter laboratory values. While your patient is taking NSAIDs, his laboratory values may reflect:

- prolonged bleeding time from suppressed platelet aggregation. Following discontinuation of NSAID therapy, effects may last less than 1 day with ibuprofen and sulindac; 2 days with tolmetin; 4 days with naproxen; and 1 week with aspirin.
- increased blood urea nitrogen (BUN) and serum creatinine concentrations.
- increased liver function test values; for example, increased serum alkaline phosphatase, serum lactic dehydrogenase, and serum transaminase concentration. With fenoprofen and sulindac, liver function tests usually return to normal despite continued use of the drug. If significant abnormalities occur, however, the doctor will discontinue the drug and possibly substitute a different NSAID.

NARCOTICS

TREATMENT FOR SEVERE PAIN

If your patient has severe pain that's not controlled by NSAIDs, the doctor may order a narcotic analgesic. By binding to opiate receptors in the central nervous system, narcotics alter both pain perception and emotional response to pain.

Unlike NSAIDs, narcotic analgesics aren't limited by a ceiling effect: in other words, narcotic analgesia continues to increase in proportion to dosage increases. However, narcotic use may be limited by the unacceptable adverse effects that accompany high dosages, including sedation and such psychotomimetic effects as hallucinations. In addition, patients using narcotics for a prolonged time develop tolerance and physical dependence.

As a nurse, you're responsible for administering narcotics as ordered. But as you know, doctor's orders may provide only dosage parameters—in many cases, you must decide exactly how much drug to give a patient.

Because of the fear of addiction and respiratory depression, you (like many of your colleagues) may be inclined to administer narcotics too conservatively. The result could be inadequate pain relief for a patient whose suffering could be easily—and safely—relieved by a higher narcotic dose.

By knowing the facts about narcotics, you'll be prepared to make the right decisions. The following information will help.

Types. Narcotics are categorized as agonists, antagonists, and mixed agonist-antagonists. Here's how they compare.

- An *agonist* mimics the activity of an endogenous substance that binds to an opiate receptor site. Narcotic agonists include morphine, heroin, hydromorphone hydrochloride (Dilaudid), codeine, oxycodone, levorphanol (Levo-Dromoran), meperidine (Demerol), propoxyphene hydrochloride (Darvon*), and methadone hydrochloride (Dolophine*).
- An *antagonist* blocks the action of an agonist drug or of the naturally occurring chemical that normally binds at the receptor site. Naloxone hydrochloride (Narcan) is considered to be a pure narcotic antagonist because it lacks opioid-like actions.
- An *agonist-antagonist* has mixed properties. In a patient who has no narcotic agonist in his system, a drug of this type acts as an agonist and causes analgesia. But if the patient already has an agonist in his system, this drug type antagonizes the agonist, reverses analgesia, and possibly causes withdrawal symptoms. As analgesics, agonist-antagonists are used primarily to manage only short-term postoperative pain because of the adverse psychotomimetic effects that develop with repeated use. Examples of agonist-antagonists include pentazocine (Talwin), nalbuphine hydrochloride (Nubain*), and butorphanol tartrate (Stadol*).

A stepped approach. To minimize the effects of drug tolerance, the doctor follows a step-up approach to pain management with narcotics. Initially, he'll order a weak narcotic agonist, such as codeine, oxycodone, or propoxyphene hydrochloride. (These drugs are also available as combination products.) If the patient develops tolerance for the drug or if his pain worsens, the doctor may increase the dosage. If this doesn't work, the doctor may then substitute a strong narcotic agonist, such as morphine, hydromorphone hydrochloride, levorphanol, meperidine, or methadone hydrochloride.

*Not available in Canada

RESPIRATORY DEPRESSION: KNOW THE FACTS

Fear of respiratory depression—realistic or not—is one of the primary reasons that many health-care professionals don't use narcotics to their full advantage. Because respiratory arrest is the cause of death for some narcotic addicts who take an overdose, the risks of respiratory depression assume exaggerated importance. Ironically, however, significant respiratory depression rarely occurs in patients who have developed tolerance to narcotics or who have acute, severe pain. Pain and emotional stress are powerful antagonists to narcotic-induced respiratory depression.

What are the risks for your patient? And how can you minimize them without diminishing analgesic effects? Read the following discussion for the answers you need.

Physiologic effects. Initially, narcotics affect respiration by decreasing the responsiveness of brain-stem regulatory centers to carbon dioxide in the blood. As a result, the patient no longer responds to respiratory drive, which is normally triggered by rising carbon dioxide blood levels. Narcotics also directly depress the pontine and medullary centers that regulate respiratory rhythm.

The onset of respiratory depression varies according to the specific drug and the route. With morphine, for example, maximal respiratory depression usually occurs within 7 minutes after I.V. administration, 30 minutes after I.M. administration, and 90 minutes after subcutaneous administration. Most narcotics cause the same degree of respiratory depression when given in equianalgesic doses.

CONTINUED ON PAGE 84

NARCOTICS CONTINUED

RESPIRATORY DEPRESSION: KNOW THE FACTS
CONTINUED

Nursing considerations. Because some degree of respiratory depression occurs even with therapeutic narcotic doses, you must monitor your patient's condition closely. Check his vital signs regularly—particularly respiratory rate, rhythm, and depth. Count his respirations for 1 minute, and observe for irregular rhythm. If the respiratory rate is 10 breaths/minute or less (or if it drops significantly below the baseline level), wake up the patient, if necessary, and ask him to breathe deeply. Assess his vital signs and mental status, and stimulate him with a position change or range-of-motion exercises.

If these measures don't improve his respiratory status and you find evidence of decreased oxygenation (for example, confusion), notify the doctor. Be prepared to administer a narcotic antagonist, such as naloxone hydrochloride (Narcan), and to provide oxygen, artificial ventilation, and other resuscitative measures if necessary.

Of course, respiratory depression isn't the only adverse effect you must guard against. For details on other adverse effects, read the information beginning on the right side of this page.

Special Note:

Patient response to a narcotic's respiratory depressant effects depends, in part, on his tolerance to the narcotic. In general, tolerance to a narcotic's respiratory depressant effects parallels tolerance to its analgesic effects.

REVERSING NARCOTIC EFFECTS WITH NALOXONE

To reverse severe narcotic-induced respiratory depression, the doctor will order naloxone—a potent narcotic antagonist. By displacing narcotics at receptor sites, naloxone reverses narcotic effects.

In addition to reversing such adverse effects as respiratory depression and sedation, naloxone reverses analgesia. It can also cause signs and symptoms of acute withdrawal after prolonged narcotic use.

Routes. Because the I.V. route permits onset of action within 2 minutes, it's the preferred route. Depending on such variables as the amount of previously administered narcotic and the naloxone dose, naloxone's effects last 15 to 90 minutes. You can also give naloxone I.M. or subcutaneously (the onset of action by these routes ranges from 2 to 5 minutes). Naloxone also has been given endotracheally in a few instances.

Note: If the patient is hypotensive or has decreased peripheral circulation, naloxone will be poorly absorbed when given I.M. or subcutaneously.

Dosage considerations. If the patient is narcotic-dependent, even a 0.4-mg I.V. bolus could precipitate withdrawal symptoms. As ordered, minimize these symptoms by diluting 0.4 mg of naloxone in 10 ml of normal saline solution and titrating it to the patient's respirations.

Since most narcotics act longer than naloxone, respiratory depression may recur. Recurrence can be prevented by a continuous infusion or repeated I.V. or I.M. injections every 1 to 2 hours.

Remember: Naloxone reverses analgesia and causes pain to return. If necessary, use other pain-relief measures.

OTHER ADVERSE EFFECTS

Respiratory depression isn't the only adverse effect to watch for when caring for a patient taking a narcotic analgesic. Monitor him for the following possible problems, and intervene as necessary.

• *Sedation.* A patient on a regular narcotic schedule may feel drowsy for the first few days after beginning therapy; however, this effect is usually temporary. Although you should expect your patient to experience some sedative effects from a narcotic, rule out other possible causes before blaming the drug. For example, the physical condition of a severely debilitated or dying patient could be responsible.

Also, don't assume that a sedated patient has obtained pain relief. If he's exhausted from continuing pain, he may be more susceptible to a narcotic's sedative effects yet remain in pain if the dosage is insufficient for analgesia.

If your patient becomes oversedated after receiving a narcotic, assess his condition and pain level. If he's not getting pain relief, the doctor should change the dosage, substitute another narcotic, or add an adjuvant (for example, an amphetamine or caffeine) to offset the narcotic's sedative effects. If the patient's pain is well controlled, the doctor may reduce the narcotic dosage.

• *Nausea and vomiting.* Most narcotics directly stimulate the medullary chemoreceptor zone and may indirectly stimulate the nearby vomiting center. Because nausea and vomiting most often afflict ambulatory patients (rather than those on bed rest), a mechanism similar to that causing motion sickness may also play a part. Apparently, narcotics have some effect on the vestibular portion of the ear, causing nausea and vomiting in conjunction with movement.

If your patient experiences nausea and vomiting after receiving a narcotic, carefully assess his condition to rule out other possible causes. Remember, continuing pain from inadequate analgesia can also cause nausea and vomiting, as can sudden hypotension.

To treat nausea and vomiting, the doctor may decrease the narcotic dosage or (if the patient is still in pain) substitute another drug. Or he may order an antiemetic (administered I.M. or rectally, if the patient is vomiting); for example, a phenothiazine, haloperidol, or hydroxyzine (Vistaril*). Symptoms will probably disappear within a week, as the patient develops tolerance to the drug.

• *Constipation.* Narcotics affect smooth muscles of the GI tract by binding to local receptor sites, increasing muscle tone. Narcotics also decrease motility, which slows gastric emptying time. As the transit time for stool is prolonged, more water is absorbed by the GI tract and the stool becomes hard and difficult to pass.

Constipation is the most common adverse effect of continuing narcotic use.

Although patients develop some tolerance to this adverse effect, those who take narcotics regularly usually have continuing problems with constipation. In general, the severity of the problem is dose-related. Every patient on continuing narcotic therapy needs a regular bowel regimen.

How narcotics affect body functions

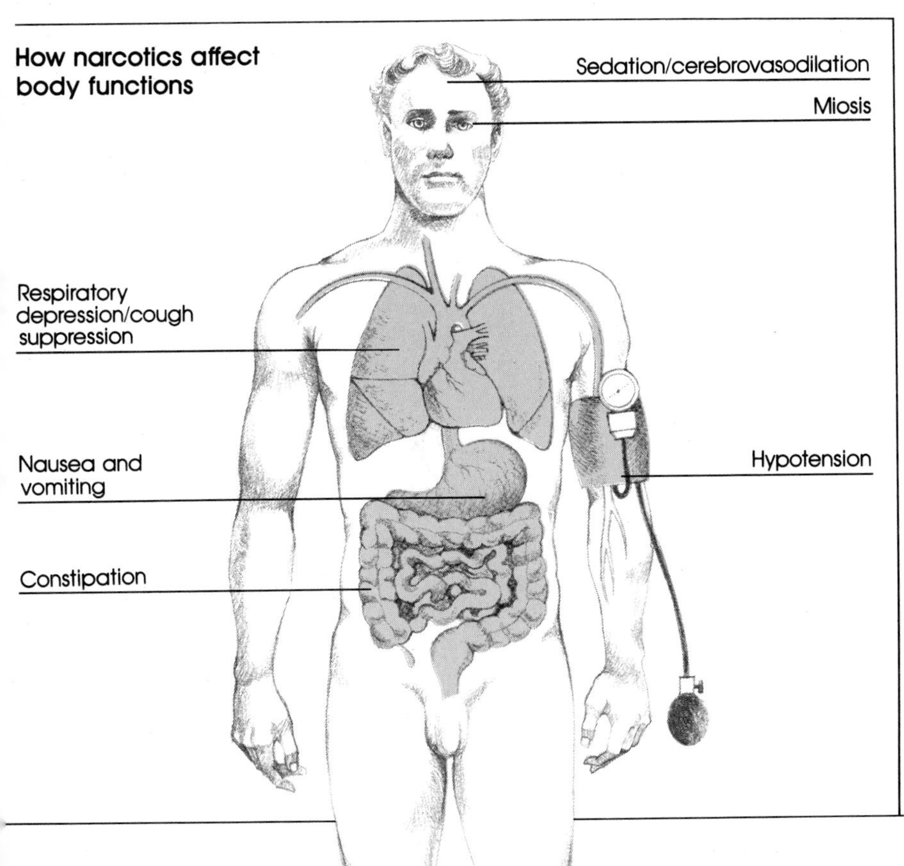

You can help your patient prevent or control constipation by recommending regular exercise and a diet high in fluids and roughage (unless contraindicated). Administer stool softeners or a peristaltic stimulant such as senna (Senokot*) as ordered. One half of a Senokot* tablet reliably reverses the constipation effect of 60 mg of codeine (or another narcotic at an equianalgesic dose). For example, if the patient is receiving 5 mg of hydromorphone hydrochloride (Dilaudid) P.O. every 4 hours, give one Senokot* tablet every 4 hours (as ordered), up to eight tablets a day. Modify the dosage according to patient response.

Note: In addition to slowing GI motility, narcotics can cause biliary tract spasm. As a result, they may be contraindicated in gallbladder disease.

• *Miosis.* A narcotic causes pupillary constriction because of its CNS effects, including a direct effect on the oculomotor nucleus.

• *Cerebrovasodilation.* This adverse effect is secondary to respiratory depression, which causes carbon dioxide levels to rise. As you know, carbon dioxide is a powerful cerebrovasodilator. Because cerebrovasodilation could elevate intracranial pressure (ICP), narcotics are contraindicated in any condition that may raise ICP (including head trauma).

• *Cough suppression.* Narcotics suppress the brain's cough center. A postoperative patient receiving narcotics needs special encouragement to cough and to deep-breathe effectively.

• *Hypotension.* Although narcotics can cause postural hypotension, they usually don't cause prolonged hypotension unless the patient is volume-depleted or has a cardiovascular condition.

*Not available in Canada

NARCOTICS CONTINUED

A CLOSER LOOK AT DRUG TOLERANCE AND DEPENDENCE

Tolerance, dependence, and addiction. What do these three words mean to you? In many cases, probably something different than what they mean to some of your colleagues. To a large extent, drug tolerance, dependence, and addiction are defined according to a person's cultural and personal values. For example, think of the patient who says with pride that he's never taken so much as an aspirin.

From a clinical standpoint, however, we can define the terms as follows:

- *Tolerance* is increased resistance to a narcotic's effects. As a patient becomes tolerant, he needs larger drug doses at more frequent intervals to achieve the desired analgesic effect. When he develops tolerance to the analgesic effects of a narcotic, he also becomes more tolerant of the drug's adverse effects, including respiratory depression and sedation.
- *Physical dependence* is an altered physiologic state produced by long-term narcotic use. Repeated use of the drug is needed to prevent withdrawal symptoms. Don't confuse tolerance and physical dependence with psychological dependence (addiction), where drug-seeking behavior is prominent irrespective of pain.
- *Addiction* has a psychological component. The addicted patient uses the drug for more than pain relief; he takes it compulsively to experience its psychic effects and perhaps to avoid withdrawal symptoms. He may or may not be physically tolerant.

Special Note:

A patient who demands a narcotic analgesic every 2 to 3 hours is probably a patient with poorly controlled pain—not a potential addict. If you encourage a patient to forego medication until pain is severe, you may inadvertently reinforce his demanding behavior and promote clock-watching. In fact, some professionals believe that such a policy can lead to psychological craving and addiction.

The development of drug addiction, which has a psychological component, is rare in medical patients with no history of addiction.

Controlling pain in an addicted patient is a problem we'll consider specifically on the next page. For now, let's focus on tolerance and dependence, two phenomena you'll encounter more frequently.

Tolerance. As a rule, the administration route determines how quickly a patient develops tolerance to a narcotic. Tolerance occurs more slowly with oral narcotic administration than with I.V. or I.M. administration. Cross-tolerance among the narcotic drugs occurs, but not completely. This means that the doctor can usually substitute one narcotic drug for another when adverse effects prevent increasing the dosage of the original drug. Because cross-tolerance isn't complete, the doctor may initially order the new narcotic at half the equianalgesic dose and then titrate the dosage according to patient response.

Dependence. Most patients become physically dependent on narcotics after using them continuously for 2 weeks or longer. To prevent signs and symptoms of withdrawal in these patients, gradually reduce the drug dosage before stopping it completely. As ordered, give one fourth of the previous 24-hour drug dose to prevent withdrawal symptoms.

Important: Physical dependence is an expected effect of narcotic therapy. Don't confuse physical dependence with psychological addiciton.

Patient teaching. If your patient is about to begin a narcotic analgesic regimen, he and his family may be concerned about the issues of physical dependence and addiction. Question them about their beliefs and concerns. Explain the difference between physical dependence and psychological addiction, and inform them that less than 1% of hospitalized patients who take narcotics for pain relief become addicted. Emphasize that physical dependence is quickly reversed after the patient no longer needs the drug for pain relief.

If the patient is still concerned about the risk of addiction, ask him a question like this: "Can you think of any reason you'd want to continue taking this drug when you no longer have pain?" If he answers *no,* reassure him that he should have little trouble discontinuing the drug when the pain subsides.

MORPHINE

CONTROLLING PAIN IN A NARCOTIC ADDICT

When you care for a patient in severe pain who's also addicted to narcotics, you face an ethical dilemma. On one hand, you may feel that you're encouraging and reinforcing his habit if you administer narcotics to control his pain. On the other hand, you know that providing pain relief is your responsibility. How do you resolve this conflict?

Perhaps by keeping in mind that you can't change an addict's behavior during one hospitalization. Your primary responsibility is to relieve his pain—and he has as much right to pain relief as any other patient. Withholding narcotics not only denies him pain relief, it could precipitate withdrawal symptoms. Also remember that, if necessary, the patient will probably find illicit ways to maintain his habit.

While caring for your patient, keep these points in mind:

- Because he has probably developed drug tolerance, he may need larger-than-normal doses to control pain. (This is true of patients on methadone maintenance as well as patients who use illicit narcotics.)
- If he's a surgical patient on methadone maintenance, discontinue oral methadone postoperatively and give parenteral doses for pain control, as ordered. After his pain subsides, the patient can return to oral methadone maintenance. Contact his methadone clinic to ensure continuity of care.
- Listen to your patient if he complains of pain. Some health-care professionals undermedicate addicted patients because of their history, denying the patients adequate pain relief.

THE PROTOTYPE NARCOTIC

Because morphine can relieve severe pain, it's the narcotic of choice for moderate-to-severe pain as well as the standard against which you compare all other narcotics.

Like other narcotics, morphine primarily affects the central nervous system (CNS) and the bowel. In addition to analgesia, morphine produces such adverse effects as respiratory depression, nausea and vomiting, sedation, mood changes, and constipation. Extremely high doses of morphine and related narcotics can also cause convulsions.

Routes. Unlike most other narcotics, morphine is effective by many administration routes. Although usually given I.V. or I.M., it can also be administered orally, rectally, sublingually, epidurally, intraventricularly, and intrathecally.

In tablet form, morphine sulfate is available at 15- and 30-mg strengths. Controlled-release tablets containing 10, 30, 60, or 100 mg of morphine sulfate are currently available in England and will soon be tested in the United States.

In liquid form, morphine sulfate is also available in doses of 10 mg/5 ml and 20 mg/5 ml. In addition, a new concentrated form of oral morphine sulfate is now available in doses of 20 mg/ml.

Morphine suppositories have been developed only recently and are available in 5-, 10-, and 20-mg sizes. They're especially useful for patients who can't take this drug orally. Before their development, oxymorphone hydrochloride (Numorphan) suppositories were used as an alternative. A 5-mg Numorphan suppository has an analgesic effect equal to that produced by 5 mg of morphine I.M.

Administering morphine by the rectal route requires a dosage adjustment. Recent evidence indicates that patients whose pain is adequately controlled on oral morphine probably won't remain pain-free if given morphine suppositories—provided the dosage remains the same. The reason: When the drug is administered rectally, the surface area available to absorb the drug is much less than when the drug is administered orally. The doctor may need to double the dosage to achieve the same pain control by the rectal route.

When changing morphine administration routes, remember that the equianalgesic dose for each route differs. *For details on equianalgesic dosage, see page 100.*

Combination products. To control pain in dying patients, morphine can be given in a combination form called Brompton's cocktail: a mixture of 15 mg morphine hydrochloride, 10 mg cocaine, 2 ml alcohol 90%, and 4 ml syrup. Schlessinger's solution, a similar mixture, consists of 1 g morphine sulfate, 2 g ethyl morphine, 12 mg scopolamine hydrochloride, and 50 ml distilled water.

In recent years, however, both Brompton's cocktail and Schlessinger's solution have been largely replaced by a simple solution of oral morphine sulfate combined with individualized adjuvant drugs, as needed. Because drug combinations are individualized according to patient response, the patient receives better pain relief.

OTHER NARCOTICS

COMPARING NARCOTICS

Narcotic analgesics fall into one of three categories: weak agonists, strong agonists, and agonist-antagonists. The following information compares commonly ordered drugs in each category. For more details about them, consult the chart beginning on page 90.

Weak agonists. Codeine, oxycodone hydrochloride, and propoxyphene hydrochloride are used for mild-to-moderate pain. They're frequently the first-line step-up approach to pain management when an NSAID is no longer effective by itself.

• *Codeine* is closely related to morphine. It has good oral efficacy: 30 mg of codeine by mouth is equianalgesic to 600 mg of aspirin in single-dose studies. Increased doses of codeine produce good analgesia, but the adverse effects of nausea, vomiting, constipation, and sedation usually prevent dosage increases. Codeine is also commonly used as an antidiarrheal and an antitussive agent.

• *Oxycodone hydrochloride,* a synthetic agent similar to morphine, is an effective short-acting analgesic. It's available as a single-entity product (Oxycodone Hydrochloride Oral Solution and Tablets*) or in combination with 325 mg of acetaminophen (Percocet**, Tylox*) or 325 mg of aspirin (Percodan). Thirty mg of oxycodone by mouth is equivalent to 10 mg of morphine by injection. However, the combination drugs contain only about 5 mg of oxycodone. Dosage increases of combination products are limited by aspirin or acetaminophen toxicity.

• *Propoxyphene hydrochloride* (Darvon*), also a synthetic agent, is structurally related to methadone and is available alone or in combination with nonnarcotic analgesic compounds.

When propoxyphene is given concurrently with carbamazepine, carbamazepine may be metabolized slowly, leading to increased blood carbamazepine levels and toxicity. Monitor a patient on both drugs for headaches, dizziness, ataxia, nausea, and fatigue.

Strong agonists. In addition to morphine, which we discussed on page 87, commonly ordered strong narcotic agonists include hydromorphone, levorphanol, meperidine, and methadone. They're effective for moderate-to-severe pain.

• *Hydromorphone hydrochloride* (Dilaudid) has a rapid onset of action similar to that of heroin. Available in oral, I.V., and rectal forms, it's an alternative to morphine (1.5 mg I.M. is equivalent to 10 mg of morphine I.M.). This short-acting narcotic is especially useful for the elderly or metabolically unstable patient.

• *Levorphanol tartrate* (Levo-Dromoran) is a highly potent synthetic narcotic with good oral efficacy. It can also be given parenterally. Its time-action curve is similar to morphine's, but it has a longer half-life. For this reason, sedative effects and confusion are greater than with morphine.

• *Meperidine hydrochloride* (Demerol) is structurally different than morphine but has similar effects. It has poor oral efficacy even though it can be administered by this route. Given parenterally, 75 mg of meperidine is equianalgesic to 10 mg of morphine. The drug is contraindicated in patients who have compromised renal function because its active, neurotoxic metabolite may accumulate and cause myoclonus and seizures.

• *Methadone hydrochloride* (Dolophine*) is a potent, long-acting narcotic analgesic with good oral efficacy. Because methadone has a long half-life (17 to 24 hours), closely watch elderly patients or those with compromised renal or hepatic function for such signs of drug accumulation as sedation and respiratory depression. Despite methadone's long half-life, you may need to administer it every 3 to 4 hours to control pain.

Chronic use of phenytoin or rifampin may increase methadone's metabolism and precipitate withdrawal symptoms. Therefore, if phenytoin or rifampin therapy is initiated or discontinued, adjust the methadone dosage as ordered.

Agonist-antagonists. These drugs aren't widely used for analgesia because of their adverse effects.

• *Pentazocine* (Talwin) in a 50-mg parenteral dose is equivalent to 10 mg of morphine I.M. Psychotomimetic effects (for example, visual hallucinations, delusions, vivid daydreams, and feelings of unreality) are common with increasing pentazocine dosages.

• *Nalbuphine hydrochloride* (Nubain*) is closely related to the pure antagonist naloxone and the narcotic agonist oxymorphone. Available for parenteral administration, it's one to two times more potent than morphine and three to five times more potent than pentazocine, with fewer psychotomimetic effects.

• *Butorphanol tartrate* (Stadol*), structurally related to pentazocine and to levorphanol, is available for parenteral administration only. As an analgesic, it's three to five times more potent than morphine.

*Not available in Canada
**Not available in the United States

DRUG UPDATE

A NEW PAIN-RELIEF OPTION

Buprenorphine hydrochloride, a partial agonist, may soon be widely available for clinical use. Because it's available in sublingual form, it offers another pain-relief option for patients who can't take oral medication.

Although similar in most respects to agonist-antagonists (such as butorphanol tartrate, nalbuphine hydrochloride, and pentazocine), buprenorphine has cardiovascular effects similar to those of morphine. However, it differs from other narcotics in several important ways:

- Compared to agonist-antagonists (particularly pentazocine), it causes few psychotomimetic effects (visual hallucinations, dysphoria, feelings of depersonalization, and nightmares).
- Compared to morphine and other agonists, it may cause slower development of tolerance and physical dependence.

Because of its antagonistic properties, buprenorphine can cause withdrawal symptoms in a patient who's recently received high or repeated doses of an agonist.

Caution: The effects of this potent drug aren't reversed by naloxone.

THE HEROIN CONTROVERSY

In the health-care community, few issues are as hotly debated as the question of whether heroin should be available for terminally ill patients in severe pain. Supporters of legalization contend that heroin acts faster and is more potent than such currently available narcotics as morphine when larger parenteral doses are required for drug-tolerant patients. Opponents, however, argue that heroin has no inherent superiority over other narcotics for these reasons:

- Heroin is a morphine derivative that the body rapidly metabolizes into morphine. Its effects in the body are the same as those of morphine, and its analgesic and adverse effects are similar.
- Heroin *is* more soluble than morphine, making it faster-acting in parenteral form. However, a new form of the synthetic narcotic hydromorphone hydrochloride—Dilaudid-HP* (high-potency)—is highly soluble. As a result, very large doses can be given in small volumes. This is important for terminally ill patients in whom the parenteral route is contraindicated.

For these reasons, heroin has no advantage over currently available narcotics. Many researchers believe that the real problem is failure of health-care professionals to administer available narcotics in dosages sufficient to control pain.

*Not available in Canada

MINIMIZING RISKS

The chart beginning on the next page provides information on commonly ordered narcotic analgesics. The following precautions apply generally when you administer any narcotic.

Contraindications

- Narcotics are usually contraindicated in patients with severe CNS depression, anoxia, hypercapnia, increased intracranial pressure, and respiratory depression (or patients at risk of respiratory depression; for example, comatose patients or those with brain tumors).
- Give narcotics with extreme caution to patients with seizure disorders, head injuries, acute alcoholism, delirium tremens, shock, myxedema, cor pulmonale, and bronchial asthma and to those with decreased respiratory reserve.

Interactions

- Narcotics combined with alcohol, phenothiazines, or tricyclic antidepressants can significantly depress the central nervous system (CNS). To minimize such effects, titrate the dosage of each to patient response, as ordered.
- Narcotics plus anticholinergics may cause severe constipation or urinary retention. Monitor the patient closely for these problems.
- Narcotics plus hydroxyzine (Vistaril*) may increase analgesia and sedation. Titrate the dosage to patient response.

NARCOTICS CONTINUED

NURSE'S GUIDE TO NARCOTIC ANALGESICS

The following chart provides guidelines for administering some narcotic analgesics. We haven't included dosage ranges because of the wide variation in patient response. As narcotic therapy progresses and the patient develops tolerance, the doctor will increase dosages.

AGONISTS

CODEINE

Onset
P.O.: 30 to 45 minutes
I.M. and *S.C.:* 10 to 30 minutes
Peak effect
P.O.: 60 to 120 minutes
I.M. and *S.C.:* 30 to 60 minutes
Duration of effect
All routes: 4 hours
Nursing considerations
• Don't administer discolored injection solution.
• Codeine may also be ordered as an antitussive or antidiarrheal.

HYDROMORPHONE HYDROCHLORIDE (Dilaudid)

Onset
P.O.: 30 minutes
I.M. and *S.C.:* 15 minutes
I.V.: 10 to 15 minutes
Rectal: Information not available
Peak effect
P.O. and *I.M.:* 30 to 90 minutes
S.C.: 15 to 30 minutes
I.V.: 30 to 90 minutes
Rectal: Information not available
Duration of effect
P.O. and *I.M.:* 4 hours
S.C.: 2 to 3 hours
I.V.: 4 hours
Rectal: Information not available
Nursing considerations
• Hydromorphone is a fast-acting, potent narcotic.
• The oral dosage form is particularly convenient for patients with chronic pain because tablets are available in 1-, 2-, 3-, and 4-mg doses.
• This drug is more likely to cause appetite loss than any other narcotic.
• Rotate injection sites to avoid induration with S.C. injections.

LEVORPHANOL TARTRATE (Levo-Dromoran)

Onset
10 to 60 minutes
Peak effect
P.O.: 90 to 120 minutes
I.M.: 60 minutes
S.C.: 60 to 90 minutes
I.V.: Within 20 minutes
Duration of effect
All routes: 4 to 8 hours
Nursing considerations
• Warn the patient that the drug has a bitter taste.
• Protect the drug from light.

MEPERIDINE HYDROCHLORIDE (Demerol)

Onset
P.O.: 15 minutes
I.M. and *S.C.:* 10 to 15 minutes
I.V.: 1 minute
Peak effect
P.O.: 60 to 90 minutes
I.M. and *S.C.:* 30 to 50 minutes
I.V.: 5 to 7 minutes
Duration of effect
All routes: 2 to 4 hours
Nursing considerations
• Meperidine may be given to patients who are allergic to morphine.
• Use the drug with extreme caution in patients with impaired renal function. Meperidine and its active metabolite normeperidine accumulate in renal failure. Closely monitor the patient for such signs of toxicity as CNS hyperirritability. Because of toxicity risks, meperidine is rarely ordered for patients with chronic cancer pain.
• Meperidine may also be given by slow I.V. infusion, preferably as a diluted solution.
• Because S.C. injections are very painful, the I.M. route is preferred.
• P.O. doses are less than half as effective as parenteral doses; give I.M., if possible.
• Give the syrup with a full glass of water. Warn the patient that the drug has a local anesthetic effect.
• Meperidine is less likely to cause smooth muscle spasm than any other narcotic; as a result, it's widely used for acute and postoperative pain. Because biliary spasm usually accompanies cholecystitis, meperidine may be ordered for pain related to this condition.

METHADONE HYDROCHLORIDE (Dolophine*)

Onset
P.O.: 30 to 60 minutes
I.M. and *S.C.:* 10 to 20 minutes
I.V.: Within 10 minutes
Peak effect
P.O.: 90 to 120 minutes
I.M. and *S.C.:* 60 to 120 minutes
I.V.: 15 to 30 minutes
Duration of effect
P.O., I.M., and *S.C.:* 4 to 6 hours
I.V.: 3 to 4 hours
Nursing considerations
• The oral dose is half as potent as the parenteral dose.
• Because S.C. injections cause local tissue irritation, the I.M. route is preferred.
• Rotate injection sites.
• The drug has a cumulative effect; marked sedation may occur with repeated doses. Use caution in elderly and debilitated patients.
• The drug is available in liquid form (1 mg/ml) for patients who can't swallow tablets. Warn the patient about its bitter taste.

*Not available in Canada

MORPHINE SULFATE

Onset
P.O.: 60 to 90 minutes
I.M. and *S.C.:* 10 to 30 minutes
I.V.: Within 10 minutes
Rectal: 60 to 90 minutes
Peak effect
P.O.: 90 to 120 minutes
I.M.: 30 to 60 minutes
S.C.: 50 to 90 minutes
I.V.: 20 minutes
Rectal: 90 to 120 minutes
Duration of effect
All routes: 4 to 5 hours
Nursing considerations
- Morphine is the drug of choice in relieving myocardial infarction pain. It may cause a transient decrease in blood pressure.
- Morphine is the drug of choice for patients with chronic cancer pain.
- Dilute the oral liquid in orange juice to improve its taste.

OXYCODONE HYDROCHLORIDE

Onset
30 minutes
Peak effect
60 minutes
Duration of effect
3 to 4 hours
Nursing considerations
- This drug is now available as a single-entity product in tablet or liquid form.
- Give the drug after meals or with milk, if possible.

OXYMORPHONE HYDROCHLORIDE (Numorphan)

Onset
I.M.: 10 to 15 minutes
S.C.: 10 to 20 minutes
I.V.: 5 to 10 minutes
Rectal: 15 to 30 minutes
Peak effect
I.M. and *S.C.:* 30 to 90 minutes
I.V.: 15 to 30 minutes
Rectal: 90 to 120 minutes
Duration of effect
I.M., S.C., and *rectal:* 3 to 6 hours
I.V.: 3 to 4 hours
Nursing consideration
- Oxymorphone is well absorbed rectally, but it's still significantly more effective if given I.M.

PROPOXYPHENE HYDROCHLORIDE (Darvon*)

Onset
15 to 60 minutes
Peak effect
120 minutes
Duration of effect
4 to 6 hours
Nursing consideration
- Propoxyphene may cause false decreases in urinary steroid excretion tests.

MIXED AGONIST-ANTAGONISTS

BUTORPHANOL TARTRATE (Stadol*)

Onset
I.M.: 10 to 30 minutes
I.V.: 2 to 3 minutes
Peak effect
I.M.: 30 to 60 minutes
I.V.: 30 minutes
Duration of effect
I.M.: 3 to 4 hours
I.V.: 2 to 4 hours
Nursing considerations
- Butorphanol is available for parenteral use only.
- The drug increases cardiac work load. Use it cautiously in patients with myocardial infarction, ventricular dysfunction, and coronary insufficiency.
- Respiratory depression doesn't increase with increased dosages, as compared to morphine at high dosages.

NALBUPHINE HYDROCHLORIDE (Nubain*)

Onset
I.M. and *S.C.:* Within 15 minutes
I.V.: 2 to 3 minutes
Peak effect
I.M. and *S.C.:* 60 minutes
I.V.: 30 minutes
Duration of effect
I.M. and *S.C.:* 3 to 6 hours
I.V.: 3 to 4 hours
Nursing considerations
- Nalbuphine is similar to pentazocine but with fewer psychotomimetic effects.
- Unlike butorphanol and pentazocine, nalbuphine doesn't increase cardiac work load.
- Respiratory depression doesn't increase with increased dosages, as compared to morphine.

PENTAZOCINE (Talwin)

Onset
P.O.: 15 to 30 minutes
I.M. and *S.C.:* 15 to 20 minutes
I.V.: 2 to 3 minutes
Peak effect
P.O.: 60 to 90 minutes
I.M. and *S.C.:* 30 to 60 minutes
I.V.: 15 to 30 minutes
Duration of effect
P.O.: 3 hours
I.M., S.C., and *I.V.:* 2 to 3 hours
Nursing considerations
- Pentazocine causes a high degree of psychotomimetic effects.
- Use caution in patients with myocardial infarction, ventricular dysfunction, and coronary insufficiency.
- The tablet form isn't well absorbed.
- Talwin-Nx*, a newly available oral form of pentazocine, contains the narcotic antagonist naloxone to prevent illicit I.V. use.

*Not available in Canada

ADJUVANT DRUGS

ANALGESIC ADJUVANTS: ATTACKING PAIN FROM ALL ANGLES

Harry Milner, a 56-year-old printer hospitalized for colon cancer, continues to complain of pain and appears restless even though he's receiving morphine 15 mg/hour by continuous I.V. infusion. Instead of increasing the morphine dosage, the doctor adds haloperidol (Haldol) to the drug regimen. The next day, Mr. Milner seems less agitated and reports that his pain's less intense. When he continues to show signs of improvement a day later, the doctor decreases the morphine dosage to 10 mg/hour.

How can a neuroleptic drug such as haloperidol help control pain? If you've cared for many patients with pain, you may know that haloperidol's just one of many analgesic adjuvants—drugs used in combination with narcotic analgesics or nonsteroidal anti-inflammatory drugs to control pain. A wide variety of drugs have been used as analgesic adjuvants. Some drugs, such as certain anticonvulsants, antihistamines (especially hydroxyzine), stimulants (for example, caffeine and dextroamphetamine), and tricyclic antidepressants, enhance analgesia. Others, such as benzodiazepines, cocaine, and most antipsychotics, can help treat adverse effects and such associated conditions as agitation.

Indications. The doctor may order an analgesic adjuvant when, for any reason, he doesn't want to increase the narcotic dosage. For example, he may believe that a higher narcotic dosage would yield only a small increase in analgesia or that a higher dosage would cause unacceptable adverse effects.

In Mr. Milner's case, the doctor chose haloperidol because it reduces agitation, which exacerbates pain.

Limitations. Adjuvants may be less effective in the following situations:

• *when your patient's narcotic dosage schedule is irregular or infrequent.* Pain tends to recur spontaneously when narcotics are administered on an as-needed basis. Before ordering an adjuvant for analgesia, the doctor should try putting the patient on a regular narcotic schedule.

• *when the patient hasn't been prepared to expect pain or hasn't been taught about its cause.* Anxiety and uncertainty can worsen pain, counteracting an adjuvant's effects. Make every effort to teach your patient about his condition and to prepare him for painful procedures.

USING CAFFEINE, CANNABINOIDS, AND COCAINE AS ADJUVANTS

Caffeine is used as an adjuvant with aspirin, acetaminophen, and salicylamide, in both over-the-counter and prescription medications. Although using these combinations is somewhat controversial, a recent study demonstrated that caffeine enhances the analgesic effects of acetaminophen, aspirin, or combinations of these drugs. The minimal effective dose of caffeine is 65 mg; the optimal dose isn't known.

Caffeine can help reduce many types of pain; for example, pain associated with oral surgery. Because caffeine improves cerebral vascular tone, it's also effective against headaches.

Cannabinoids, substances derived from the hemp plant, may act as euphorics, analgesics, appetite stimulants, and most effectively as antiemetics. Marijuana, a cannabis derivative, is under investigation as an antiemetic; however, its future use may be limited because of such adverse effects as drowsiness, hypotension, bradycardia, and dysphoria (particularly in the elderly).

Cocaine is most commonly used as a local and regional anesthetic for oral and nasal mucosa. It seems to lack specific analgesic properties, although it can improve a patient's alertness. Elderly patients given a mixture of cocaine and morphine may experience restlessness, agitation, and confusion.

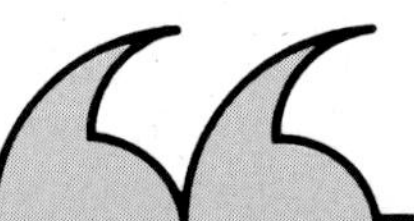

"Adjuvants shouldn't be used indiscriminately. Most of them increase the sedative effects of narcotics, which may prevent the doctor from raising the narcotic dosage sufficiently for pain control. Adjuvants are best added after narcotic dosages are titrated for optimum analgesia."

Richard Payne, MD
Assistant Attending Neurologist
Memorial Sloan-Kettering
Cancer Center
New York

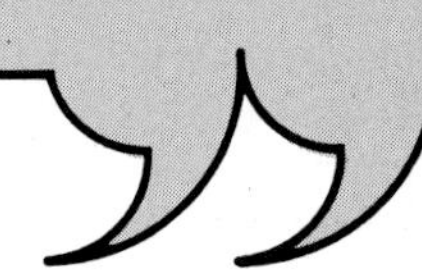

MATCHING ADJUVANTS TO PAIN-RELATED SYMPTOMS

Which drug would the doctor choose if he's considering an analgesic adjuvant for your patient? That depends on the patient's symptoms and clinical condition.

An adjuvant is most effective when the target is a specific symptom—either pain or another symptom contributing to pain. Read the chart below for details about indications, dosages, and nursing considerations for drugs ordered most frequently as analgesic adjuvants.

Important: These dosage ranges are guidelines only. Adjust dosages appropriately (as ordered), according to patient response.

ANTICONVULSANTS

CARBAMAZEPINE (Tegretol)

Dosage and route
600 to 1,200 mg/day P.O. in three or four divided doses

Indication
Neuralgic pain (especially trigeminal neuralgia)

Nursing considerations
- Tell the doctor immediately if signs and symptoms of blood dyscrasias occur; for example, fever, mouth ulcers, sore throat, and bruising.
- Tell the patient to expect mild-to-moderate sedation or dizziness when he begins taking the drug. This effect usually disappears in 3 to 4 days.
- Monitor the patient for ataxia and drowsiness when giving carbamazepine with a narcotic analgesic.

CLONAZEPAM (Clonopin*, Rivotril)

Dosage and route
1 to 6 mg/day P.O.

Indication
Neuralgic pain

Nursing considerations
- This drug is contraindicated in patients with closed-angle glaucoma.
- Monitor the patient for oversedation.
- Never withdraw the drug suddenly.

ANTIHISTAMINES

HYDROXYZINE (Atarax, Vistaril*)

Dosage and route
25 to 400 mg/day P.O. or I.M. before bed or in divided doses

Indications
Nausea, mild anxiety

Nursing considerations
- When giving the drug I.M., insert the needle deep into a large muscle.
- Suggest sugarless hard candy or gum to relieve dry mouth.
- Monitor the patient for excessive sedation.

ANTIPSYCHOTICS

CHLORPROMAZINE (Chlorzine*, Thorazine*)

Dosage and route
10 to 600 mg/day P.O., I.V., I.M., or by rectal suppository before bed or in three or four divided doses

Indications
Anxiety, nausea or vomiting from narcotic, need for sedation

Nursing considerations
- Document the patient's baseline blood pressure measurements before beginning therapy.
- When giving the drug I.M., insert the needle deep in the upper outer quadrant of the buttocks only. Slowly massage the site afterward to prevent a sterile abscess. *Note:* The injection stings.
- Monitor the patient's blood pressure regularly throughout therapy, and watch for orthostatic hypotension. After parenteral administration, keep the patient supine for 1 hour and advise him to rise slowly.
- Protect the oral liquid form from light. (A yellowish color change is common and doesn't affect potency.)
- Dilute the oral liquid form with fruit juice, milk, or semisolid food just before administration.
- Monitor the patient for severe extrapyramidal reactions. Keep diphenhydramine (Benadryl) handy to treat such reactions.

FLUPHENAZINE (Permitil*, Prolixin*)

Dosage and route
3 to 20 mg/day P.O. or I.M. before bed or in two divided doses

Indications
Anxiety, need for increased analgesia (especially in trigeminal neuralgia, postherpetic neuralgia, and diabetic neuropathy)

Nursing considerations
- Protect the oral liquid form from light. (A yellowish color change is common and doesn't affect potency.)

*Not available in Canada

CONTINUED ON PAGE 94

ADJUVANT DRUGS CONTINUED

MATCHING ADJUVANTS TO PAIN-RELATED SYMPTOMS
CONTINUED

FLUPHENAZINE continued

• Dilute the oral liquid form with water, fruit juice, milk, or semisolid food just before administration.
• Monitor the patient for severe extrapyramidal reactions. Keep diphenhydramine (Benadryl) handy to treat such reactions.

HALOPERIDOL (Haldol)

Dosage and route
1 to 20 mg/day P.O. or I.M. before bed or in two divided doses

Indications
Anxiety, nausea, hallucinations associated with an analgesic drug

Nursing considerations
• Protect the oral liquid form from light. (A yellowish color change is common and doesn't affect potency.)
• Monitor the patient for severe extrapyramidal reactions. Keep diphenhydramine (Benadryl) handy to treat such reactions.

BENZODIAZEPINES

DIAZEPAM (Valium)

Dosage and route
5 to 40 mg/day P.O. before bed or in three or four divided doses

Indications
Muscle spasm or myoclonic jerks, anxiety, insomnia

Nursing considerations
• Avoid giving the drug I.M.
• Monitor the patient for oversedation.

STIMULANTS

DEXTROAMPHETAMINE METHYLPHENIDATE HYDROCHLORIDE (Ritalin)

Dosage and route
10 to 40 mg/day P.O. in morning

Indications
Somnolence, lethargy

Nursing considerations
• This drug may be habit-forming.
• Closely monitor the patient for hypertension and excessive stimulation. *Note:* He may become fatigued as the drug effects wear off.
• Tell him to avoid caffeine.

TRICYCLIC ANTIDEPRESSANTS

AMITRIPTYLINE (Elavil, Endep*) DOXEPIN (Adapin*, Sinequan) IMIPRAMINE HYDROCHLORIDE (Tofranil)

Dosage and route
25 to 300 mg/day P.O. before bed or in two divided doses

Indications
Insomnia, depression, pain from trigeminal neuralgia, neuropathies (especially diabetic neuropathy), postherpetic neuralgia, migraine headache

Nursing considerations
• Check the patient for urinary retention and constipation. Increase his fluid intake to lessen constipation. Suggest a stool softener, if needed.
• Prepare him for initial drowsiness, which usually wears off.
• Suggest sugarless hard candy or gum to relieve dry mouth.

*Not available in Canada

PLACEBOS

PRESCRIPTION: PLACEBO

The doctor orders a placebo for Lillian Strayer, age 44, when he can't locate the source of her abdominal pain. Do you know why he wants you to administer it? How do you feel about giving Mrs. Strayer a medication with no active ingredient or intrinsic therapeutic value? If she responds positively to the placebo, will you conclude that her pain was imaginary?

Like many nurses, you may have misconceptions about why placebos are used and how they work. And you may worry about the ethical, moral, and legal implications of administering them. You need to know where you stand on these issues. Then you'll be prepared to dispel myths about placebos, decide whether to administer them, and use your knowledge to enhance pain-control measures.

Defining placebos. A placebo is any medical treatment or nursing measure that works because of its implicit or explicit therapeutic *intent* rather than its chemical or physical properties. A placebo is usually a capsule containing lactose or an injection of saline solution, although it can be virtually anything. For example, one patient, unfamiliar with the purpose of electrocardiography, reported that an EKG relieved his chest pain.

Even surgery can have a placebo effect. In one study, patients who'd undergone internal mammary artery implantation for angina pain reported the surgery reduced their pain by 60% to 90% regardless of whether the artery remained patent—suggesting that surgery had a placebo effect.

DISPELLING MYTHS ABOUT PLACEBOS

Myths and misconceptions about placebos die hard. The following checklist presents some common myths and their implications for patient care.

- **Myth:** *Placebos can be used to distinguish "real" pain of physical origin from psychogenic pain (not of physical origin, thus not requiring active treatment).* All pain is real to the patient who has it. However, some doctors and nurses have mistakenly used placebos to determine if a patient's pain is "real" or to prove that a patient's exaggerating or faking his symptoms. But a positive placebo response doesn't prove or disprove the origin of a patient's pain. Studies show that placebos *can* relieve pain from obvious physical stimuli (for example, a surgical wound).
- **Myth:** *Placebos won't reduce severe pain.* In some cases, they can. In a double-blind study of patients with chronic, moderate-to-severe pain from cancer, about 77% of patients obtained pain relief from placebos.
- **Myth:** *Pain relief from a placebo suggests that anxiety is the major component of the patient's pain; thus, placebos must have a psychological rather than physical effect.* Many doctors mistakenly believe placebos don't affect physiologic function. However, placebos can produce objectively measurable physiologic effects. For example, a doctor administered ipecac syrup, an emetic, to a patient with a gastric fistula, telling her the drug would *relieve* her nausea. Within 15 minutes, her nausea disappeared and the gastric atony that accompanies nausea was replaced by normal gastric peristalsis. Obviously the ipecac placebo had produced an unexpected physiologic change.

  Although not all placebos are physiologically active, they've also been shown to increase serum hydrocortisone levels, decrease serum lipid levels, and cause eosinophilia and anaphylactic reactions.
- **Myth:** *Placebos are harmless and have no adverse effects.* Since placebos can cause physiologic changes, they're potentially harmful. Common adverse effects of placebos include nausea, vomiting, and upset stomach.
- **Myth:** *Patients who respond to placebos are unintelligent or neurotic.* Because such a patient has been, in a sense, fooled, some health-care professionals conclude that he must be unintelligent or emotionally unstable. However, research shows that the more educated the patient, the more likely he'll respond to a placebo.

  A more accurate conclusion about this patient is that he's highly motivated to obtain pain relief and receptive to anything or anyone that might help.
- **Myth:** *Because placebos aren't active drugs, a nurse can administer them without doctor's orders.* Wrong. A nurse can't legally administer a placebo without doctor's orders.
- **Myth:** *A placebo won't work if the patient knows he may be receiving one.* In one instance, a few patients who were told they were receiving a placebo continued to take it for weeks and in some cases months, claiming it relieved their pain. Placebos have also been effective for patients taking part in double-blind studies, in which neither the patient nor the nurse knows whether the medication given is the placebo or an active ingredient.

HOW PLACEBOS WORK

Hundreds of studies show that placebos reduce pain, relieve allergies, clear skin blemishes, decrease blood pressure, and treat bleeding ulcers. Placebos frequently have the same onset, time of peak effect, and duration of action as the analgesics with which they're being compared.

However, pain relief can't always be attributed to the placebo's action. For example, a patient who's given a placebo after receiving analgesics over a long period may improve from the cumulative analgesic effect, not from the placebo. And in some cases, pain relief results from spontaneous, normally occurring fluctuations in pain intensity. In other words, pain relief is a coincidence.

But many patients experience pain reduction from the placebo itself. What causes a true, positive placebo response? For some patients, placebos may work by reducing anxiety. Some studies suggest that placebos rarely relieve pain in patients who aren't anxious.

Classical conditioning may also play a part in a true placebo response. For instance, a patient who's been receiving morphine injections may associate the injection procedure with pain relief and respond positively to an injection of saline solution if he believes it's morphine.

Finally, some researchers propose a biochemical mechanism, theorizing that the expectation of pain relief stimulates the production of endorphins, the body's natural pain-relieving substances.

PLACEBOS CONTINUED

WHO RESPONDS TO PLACEBOS?

Although not every patient will respond to a placebo, research shows that roughly one out of every three patients can obtain some degree of pain relief from placebo medication. A patient who responds positively is called a *placebo reactor.* Most placebo reactors respond positively only under certain conditions. Very few patients *always* respond to placebos.

Placebo reactors usually respond only for a few days or at most a few weeks. However, some patients who have received analgesics for long periods can be maintained on placebos. And some patients continue to benefit from a placebo even when told they're taking one.

Since many patients will respond favorably to a placebo at some time, outstanding characteristics of placebo reactors are hard to identify. But a recent study using easily observable personal data showed that most reactors fall into one or more of the following categories:
- widower or divorcé
- single or married woman with children
- farmer or professional
- college graduate
- nonsmoker.

Placebo reactors didn't significantly differ from nonreactors in terms of gender, age, number of siblings, alcohol consumption, or history of physical or emotional illness. The researchers concluded from these findings that placebo reactors tend to have many responsibilities and little opportunity to indulge in the dependency that pain and illness usually cause.

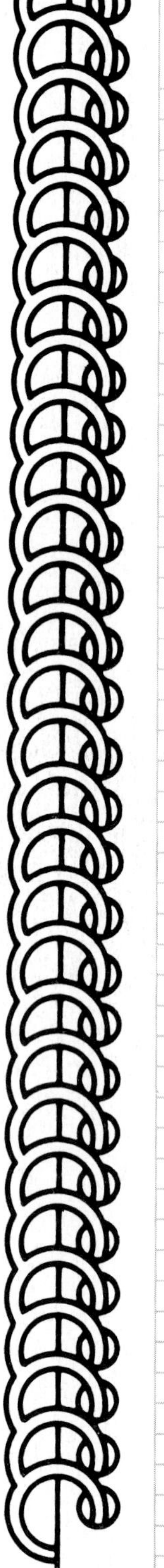

CRITICAL QUESTIONS

PLACEBOS AND PROFESSIONAL ETHICS

A placebo order opens a Pandora's box of ethical and moral issues. The following questions can help you decide how and when to administer a placebo.

- *Can you legally administer a placebo?* Yes, provided the doctor has written an order.
- *Why is a placebo being considered?* Make sure you understand the placebo's purpose.
- *Will the doctor obtain informed consent?* Informed consent isn't legally necessary. But if you don't tell the patient what you're giving him, you may feel you're deceiving him. To avoid this situation, ask the doctor to order a drug regimen that alternates an active analgesic with the placebo. The hospital pharmacy can set up a code so that the placebo and the active drug can be administered using the double-blind method. Explain the plan to the patient, and ask for his consent.
- *If the doctor doesn't obtain informed consent, how will you respond when your patient finds out he's been given a placebo?* Will he lose his trust in you? If you don't want to risk losing your patient's trust, don't administer a placebo without first obtaining informed consent and using the double-blind method.
- *Can you refuse to administer a placebo?* Suppose the doctor hasn't obtained informed consent and isn't using the double-blind method. Do you feel uncomfortable deceiving your patient? Legally, you can refuse to administer the placebo if you believe it could harm the patient. Harm may include jeopardizing the nurse-patient relationship. If you decide not to give a placebo, document this in the patient's chart and notify your supervisor and the doctor.
- *If you decide to give the placebo, even though the patient isn't informed about it, how will you respond if he asks you about his medication?* Decide how you'll answer his questions *before* you administer a placebo. You may decide to make up a name for the placebo. But if you don't want to lie to him, refer him to the doctor—or tell him the truth. If you do so, document this in the patient's chart and tell the doctor at once. Protect the patient from getting conflicting information from staff members.

ANALGESIC GUIDELINES

[C]REATING A POSITIVE [P]LACEBO ENVIRONMENT

[H]ow a placebo's presented to a [p]atient can play a crucial role [i]n his response. The following [f]actors promote patient accep[t]ance:

Convincing stimuli. Elaborate [e]quipment, a long series of pro[c]edural steps, parenteral rather [t]han oral administration, and de[t]ailed explanations have the [g]reatest impact. The more con[v]incing the stimuli, the more [l]ikely the placebo response will [b]e positive.

Administration by a trusted ex[p]ert. Faith is important in the [p]lacebo response. Your confi[d]ence in the treatment and your [s]kill in implementing it contribute [t]o a positive response. By the [s]ame token, if the patient senses [t]hat you're skeptical about the [t]reatment, he's less likely to re[s]pond positively.

Note: Reinforcing the patient's [t]rust in his doctor also helps build [c]onfidence in the placebo.

• *Focusing attention on the pain.* When you administer the medi[c]ation, make sure to tell the pa[t]ient it's for pain relief. Letting [h]im know you're doing something [t]o reduce his pain increases the [c]hance of a positive response.

• *Explaining the placebo's intent.* Tell the patient that the medication should make him feel better. You might want to go even one step further, saying, "This has helped many patients with pain like yours" or "This is one of the best ways to relieve your pain."

Even the suggestion that a placebo will reduce pain—for instance, by giving an injection in response to a pain complaint—may be enough to elicit a positive response.

IDEAL ANALGESIA: AN ELUSIVE GOAL

Most patients in pain depend on analgesic drugs for relief. But which analgesic is safest and most effective for *your* patient? How much of it should you administer?

Don't assume the doctor will always make these decisions. In many cases, his orders provide only guidelines. For example, the doctor may let you choose from among several different analgesics. And for each, he may give only a dosage range, expecting you to titrate the dose as necessary. In some cases, he may even let you choose from among two or more administration routes.

To make the right decisions, rely on your assessment skills. Your goal? To provide optimum pain relief with the fewest possible adverse effects.

Start by assessing the severity of your patient's pain. Determine when his pain occurs, when it's mildest, and when it's most severe.

Then check his chart for information on previous analgesic use. Which analgesics has he received in the past? At what dosage? How long did pain relief last?

Also note his age, since this can affect drug metabolism. In general, patients between ages 18 and 29 need more frequent doses than patients over age 30. Elderly patients may need less frequent analgesic doses than do middle-aged patients for the same degree of pain relief. Elderly patients may also experience excessive sedation and respiratory depression from repeated doses of drugs with long half-lives, such as methadone. They're likely to experience fewer adverse effects from drugs with shorter half-lives, such as hydromorphone hydrochloride (Dilaudid).

HOW DRUG COMBINATIONS ENHANCE ANALGESIA

To assess your patient's pain, use your assessment findings and ask him to rate his pain on a 0-to-10 scale. As ordered, you'll probably give a narcotic analgesic for severe acute pain or a nonsteroidal anti-inflammatory drug for mild pain. But if your patient doesn't get adequate pain relief from one drug type, combining drugs is an option that may provide relief without increasing the risks of raising the narcotic dosage.

Why does this combination enhance analgesia? Because narcotics and NSAIDs have different mechanisms of action: narcotics act mainly on the central nervous system, NSAIDs mainly on the peripheral nervous system. In combination, these drugs block pain at two levels.

When administering a combination product, such as Percodan, don't assume that it automatically produces additive analgesia. Although such a product contains a nonnarcotic (aspirin) in addition to the narcotic, the nonnarcotic dose is usually the equivalent of only a single aspirin tablet. Supplement a narcotic compound tablet with one or two aspirin or acetaminophen tablets.

If your patient's receiving narcotics I.M., he could still benefit from an oral nonnarcotic added to his regimen—assuming, of course, that he can tolerate oral medications. If he can't, consider giving aspirin or acetaminophen in a rectal suppository. Keep in mind, however, that rectal absorption is unreliable, so closely monitor patient response.

Note: Because aspirin and acetaminophen are antipyretics, they're contraindicated when they could mask fever.

ANALGESIC GUIDELINES CONTINUED

P.R.N. OR AROUND THE CLOCK: CHOOSING THE RIGHT DOSAGE SCHEDULE

To determine whether your patient should receive an analgesic p.r.n. or around the clock (a.t.c.), use the following questions as a guide:
- Is the patient's pain acute or chronic?
- How long has he been receiving the medication?
- Does he have an uncontrolled metabolic disorder (for example, diabetes or metabolic acidosis or alkalosis)?

In general, give medication p.r.n. if your patient is metabolically unstable of if he has acute intermittent pain from surgery or a therapeutic or diagnostic procedure. But don't wait until pain becomes severe to administer analgesics, particularly if your patient has just had surgery. Severe pain can slow his recovery by limiting his movement, coughing, and deep breathing. To prevent pain from becoming severe, administer medication as soon as pain begins—or even sooner, if you anticipate that he'll have pain.

Preventing severe pain is easier than relieving it—and usually requires a lower analgesic dosage.

If your patient has chronic pain (for example, from cancer), administer analgesics p.r.n. for 24 to 48 hours. Once pain relief is achieved, the doctor will calculate the patient's analgesic requirements over a 24-hour period. Administer the calculated total in divided doses at fixed intervals a.t.c. or as a continuous infusion, as ordered.

To prevent severe pain from recurring, keep dosage intervals short and regularly assess your patient's pain. If your patient with cancer is scheduled for a.t.c medication, awaken him throughout the night, as necessary, to give the analgesic.

Note: If your patient's receiving methadone, the doctor may specify p.r.n. administration to avoid the drug's cumulative adverse effects.

ADMINISTRATION ROUTE CONSIDERATIONS

When determining which administration route is best for your patient, consider his prognosis as well as the nature and severity of his pain. For example, a postoperative patient will probably need I.M. analgesics only for a few days; then, he can be switched to the oral route.

If your patient is dying and has chronic pain, use the oral route as long as possible. When the oral route is no longer appropriate (for example, because he can't tolerate anything by mouth) and he needs frequent analgesic injections, consider such alternatives as rectal administration, continuous subcutaneous infusion, or intermittent (or continuous) I.V. infusion. For more about infusion therapy, see the information beginning on page 102.

Also take into account how a particular administration route influences the analgesic drug's onset of action and duration of effect. For example, if your patient has acute pain and needs immediate relief, he'll benefit most from parenteral administration. Drugs given I.V. have the fastest onset of action, producing analgesia in 10 to 15 minutes. But keep in mind that drugs given I.V. have the shortest duration of effect, so you may have to administer them at 1- to 2-hour intervals.

When administering I.M. analgesics, choose the injection site carefully. Studies show that when morphine and methadone are injected into the deltoid muscle, they take effect more rapidly and give greater pain relief than when they're injected into the gluteal muscle.

Note: After surgery, drugs given I.M. may be poorly absorbed. If your postoperative patient isn't getting pain relief from I.M. analgesics, increase the dosage or change the route, as ordered.

When parenteral administration is contraindicated and the patient can't take oral medication (for example, because he's vomiting) administer drugs via the rectal route, if possible. Oxymorphone hydrochloride (Numorphan), for example, is well absorbed rectally; it's an alternative to narcotics with more limited dosage forms. But most drugs are irregularly or incompletely absorbed by the rectal route. Administer larger doses, as ordered, and monitor patient response.

Note: In general, the rectal route is contraindicated when the patient has a disorder affecting the lower GI tract; for example, rectal bleeding or diarrhea.

RULE OF ThumB

When changing from the I.M. or subcutaneous route to the I.V. route, give an I.V. dose that's half the I.M. or subcutaneous dose. Then, titrate the dosage up or down, according to patient response.

ASSESSING YOUR PATIENT'S DRUG THERAPY

Once you've decided on an appropriate analgesic regimen, you'll need to assess its effectiveness. Observe your patient's response to the initial analgesic dose. Then ask yourself these questions:

• *Is your patient receiving adequate analgesia? Is he oversedated?* If the analgesic relieves his pain but oversedates him or significantly decreases his respiratory rate, the dose is probably too high. So before you begin administering the medication, document the patient's respiratory rate and level of consciousness for later comparison. (A flow sheet can help you identify trends.) Consider that sedation usually occurs before any significant respiratory depression, so closely observe the sedated patient for changes in respiratory function.

Don't confuse normal sleep with undesirable analgesic-induced sedation. If you have trouble distinguishing the two, closely observe your patient's respiratory function every ½ hour. If respiration seems satisfactory, wait to see what effect the next dose has. If the patient is drowsy after the second dose, ask the doctor to reduce the dosage or to change the drug if necessary for pain control.

• *Is the patient receiving too little analgesic?* If he's receiving medication I.M. or subcutaneously, the dose is probably too low if he still has significant pain 1 to 1½ hours after the injection. Maximum pain relief should occur within that time.

• *Is the choice of analgesic appropriate?* If your patient's sedated but still has pain, you may need to give smaller doses more frequently or substitue a shorter-acting drug. Don't assume your patient's pain is under control simply because he's asleep or sedated. A patient whose pain has kept him awake or made him restless may doze off after receiving an analgesic dose that only partially relieves his pain. His drowsiness results from fatigue.

• *Is the interval between doses too long?* Suspect this if most of your patient's pain returns before his next scheduled dose or if he becomes a clock watcher. Parenteral analgesics usually relieve pain for 3 to 4 hours and in some cases up to 6 hours (except those given I.V., because duration of action is shorter by this route). In some cases, an analgesic such as hydromorphone hydrochloride (Dilaudid) may be given by injection at 2- to 3-hour intervals to relieve pain. This drug has a rapid onset of action (15 to 30 minutes after I.M. injection), so it's particularly effective for acute pain.

HOW TO MODIFY ANALGESIC THERAPY

Suppose the analgesic you're administering doesn't relieve your patient's pain. Or it does relieve his pain but not fast enough or only for short periods. What's your next step?

If doctor's orders permit, increase the dosage or administer the drug more frequently. If these measures don't help, consider changing the administration route or switching to a different drug.

If you must change the drug or the administration route, calculate the new dosage carefully to ensure that it's at least *equianalgesic* to the first drug. Drugs given in equianalgesic dosages produce the same analgesic effect.

Changing the administration route. Refer to an equianalgesic chart like the one on page 100 when changing a drug's administration route. However, be aware that equianalgesic doses may vary from one patient to the next.

If your patient's been receiving an I.M. or I.V. analgesic, he may become anxious if the drug is switched to an oral route, especially if he's previously had inadequate pain relief from oral analgesics. Consequently, never change routes abruptly. Instead, convert half the I.V. or I.M. dose to the equivalent P.O. dose, and give both simultaneously. Over the next few days, decrease the I.M. or I.V. dose while increasing the P.O. dose until the patient is receiving only P.O. medication and getting adequate pain relief. *Note:* During this transition period, ask the doctor for a p.r.n. analgesic order in case the P.O. dose doesn't adequately relieve your patient's pain.

When changing from one narcotic analgesic to another, administer the new narcotic in a dosage that's about one half to two thirds of the first drug's dosage. Then titrate the dosage according to patient response.

Ending analgesic therapy. When your patient no longer has pain, he'll no longer need an analgesic. But if he's been receiving a narcotic regularly for 2 weeks or longer, he may have developed physical dependence on the drug. If you eliminate the drug abruptly, he may have withdrawal symptoms. To prevent withdrawal, reduce the narcotic dosage about 25% every day or two, depending on his reaction, until you've completely eliminated the drug.

ANALGESIC GUIDELINES CONTINUED

COMPARING ANALGESIC POTENCIES

The chart below shows equianalgesic dosages for drugs commonly used to treat patients with moderate-to-severe pain. Use the chart as a guideline when changing your patient's drug or administration route.

Note: Morphine is used as a standard for comparison.

ANALGESIC	DOSAGE (mg)				EQUIVALENT MORPHINE DOSAGE (mg I.M.)
	S.C./I.M.	P.O.	I.V.	RECTAL	
Nonnarcotics					
acetaminophen (Tempra, Tylenol)		650		300 to 650†	2
aspirin		650		300 to 650†	
Narcotics					
butorphanol tartrate (Stadol*)	2		1		10
codeine	130	200			10
hydromorphone hydrochloride (Dilaudid)	1.5	7.5	1		10
levorphanol tartrate (Levo-Dromoran)	2	4	1		10
meperidine hydrochloride (Demerol)	75	300	50		10
methadone hydrochloride (Dolophine*)	10	20	5		10
morphine sulfate	10	30††	5		10
nalbuphine hydrochloride (Nubain*)	10		5		10
oxycodone hydrochloride		30			10
oxymorphone hydrochloride (Numorphan)	1		0.5	10	10
pentazocine (Talwin)	60	180			10

*Not available in Canada
†Inconsistently absorbed; dose must be titrated for each patient.
††For chronic dosing only. For single dosing, give 60 mg.

FOR THE PATIENT

TAKING MEDICATION

The nurse has explained how to take your pain medication properly. Use this aid as a reminder of what you've learned when you go home.

Take your medication regularly, as directed by the doctor. Don't try to wait until you're in a lot of pain, or you may have trouble controlling the pain.

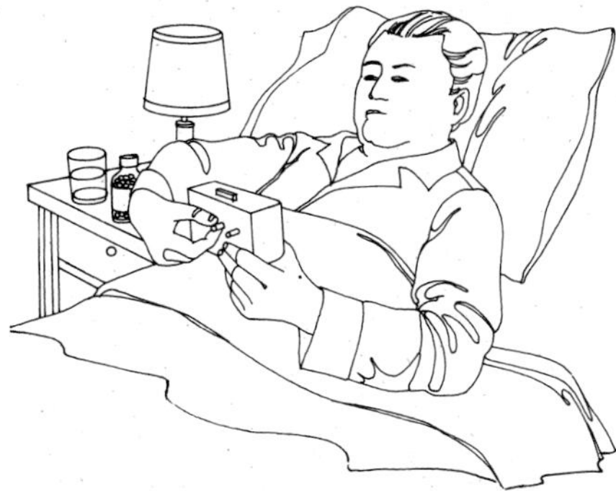

If your pain is particularly bad when you wake up in the morning, the reason may be that you didn't have enough medication in your bloodstream to last the night. To help, take your medication one or more times *during* the night, as needed, at the same dosage intervals you follow during the day. For example, if you take medication every 4 hours and you go to bed at 10 p.m., set your alarm for 2 a.m. and take another dose. If necessary, reset your alarm for 6 a.m. and take still another dose then.

If you've been taking medication for 2 weeks or longer, don't suddenly stop taking it without the doctor's consent—even if you no longer have pain. Your body may have become used to the medication you're taking. If you suddenly stop taking it, you may have unpleasant or dangerous adverse effects. Check with the doctor for guidelines.

At some time, you may notice that the pain medication you have been taking no longer seems to work as well as it did. If this happens, call your doctor so he can find new ways to control your pain.

Also call the doctor if:
- the medication he's prescribed makes you feel sleepy or less alert.
- you develop a new pain or your pain seems different.
- you become constipated during treatment. Follow the doctor's suggestions about modifying your diet, drinking extra fluids, and taking a mild laxative.

DEALING WITH CONSTIPATION

If you're taking a narcotic medication, it may make you constipated. Here are some guidelines to help:
- Eat more high-fiber foods, including raw fruits and vegetables, whole grain breads and cereals, dried fruits, and nuts. Choose high-fiber snack foods such as date-nut bread, oatmeal cookies, or granola. Add 1 to 2 tablespoons of bran to your cereal or eggs.
- Drink warm or hot beverages to stimulate bowel activity.
- Avoid hard cheeses and refined grain products, such as rice and macaroni.
- Get more exercise (for example, walking) if you can.

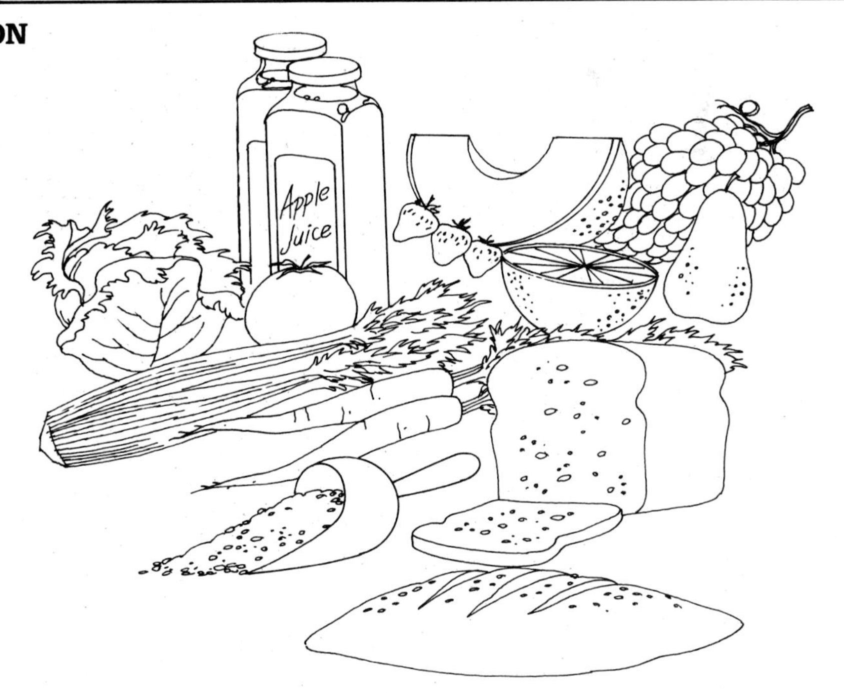

SPECIAL INFUSION SYSTEMS

INFUSION SYSTEMS: REFINING DRUG DELIVERY

Ada Benson, age 52, has severe, continuous pain from advanced colon cancer. She has an intestinal obstruction, so you can't give her oral analgesics. And because of the amount of drug she needs for pain relief, the rectal route isn't practical. That's why you've been administering 15 mg of morphine I.M. every 3 hours. But the injections have made her skin sclerotic, increasing her pain.

How can you help relieve Mrs. Benson's pain consistently while minimizing complications? Suggest that the doctor consider a continuous subcutaneous or I.V. infusion for morphine administration. By delivering medication continuously, infusion therapy provides steady pain control. In addition, the patient may get relief from a lower total drug dosage.

Infusion therapy eliminates trauma and complications associated with multiple I.M. or subcutaneous injections. By providing steady pain control, a continuous infusion may also reduce the anxiety associated with pain.

I.V. morphine infusion. If the doctor orders I.V. infusion therapy for your patient with severe, chronic pain, chances are he'll choose morphine as the medication. During therapy, monitor your patient frequently for adverse reactions, particularly increased sedation, respiratory depression, and confusion.

To avoid problems, monitor your patient's level of consciousness, respiratory status, and vital signs at least every 4 hours (or more frequently, if indicated). Titrate the dosage as ordered for maximum pain relief with minimal adverse effects. If his respiratory rate falls below 10 breaths/minute (or significantly below the baseline level), notify the doctor. Stay with the patient and monitor his respiratory rate. Try stimulating him by waking him and repositioning him. If his respiratory rate continues to drop despite intervention, be prepared to discontinue the morphine infusion.

Important: As with any narcotic, keep naloxone handy to reverse respiratory depression, if necessary.

Other infusion routes. Previously, only hospitalized patients could receive infusion therapy—and then only by the I.V. route. But now, more advanced infusion systems, designed for both hospital and outpatient use, can deliver morphine and other analgesics by other routes as well; for example, subcutaneously, intraventricularly, intrathecally, and epidurally.Some systems are portable; others are implantable. With some patient-controlled infusion devices, the patient can use the pump as often as he needs to—up to a preset limit determined by the doctor. (For details read the chart at right.)

Any patient who goes home with a continuous subcutaneous or epidural morphine infusion system must live with a family member or friend who has been taught to monitor the patient for excessive sedation and respiratory depression. The patient also needs consistent follow-up by a health-care professional who's available to answer questions and give advice at any time, day or night.

Special Note:

Always administer a continuous narcotic infusion with a microdrip I.V. set and an infusion pump.

COMPARING A FEW INFUSION SYSTEMS

Drug infusion systems deliver drugs either continuously or intermittently. To compare the features, benefits, and drawbacks of several infusion systems, study the chart below.

Keep in mind that infusion systems are relatively new as pain-control aids. The doctor will try other methods before ordering an infusion system for analgesia. For more information on using these systems, contact a hospital that specializes in cancer treatment where these systems may be in use for cancer chemotherapy or pain relief.

Important: Maintain aseptic technique when handling equipment.

CORMED INFUSION PUMP SYSTEM

Designed to allow the patient ambulation during treatment, this system includes a power pack, a pump, a 40- to 60-cc drug reservoir bag, and an adjustable flow meter. It can provide continuous analgesic infusion by several possible routes: I.V. (via a peripheral or central catheter) or subcutaneous (through a 27G pediatric wing-tip needle taped in place).

Advantages

- Portable
- Attaches easily to a specially designed shoulder harness or belt
- Contains a sterile medication bag and tubing set within the pump case, minimizing the risk of contamination
- Has a rechargeable power pack that lasts for 100 charges, or about 2 years
- Has an adjustable flow rate
- Power-pack charger and plug-in flow-rate meter allow precise flow-rate adjustment

Disadvantages
• System weighs almost 2 lb (9.5 kg); it may be too heavy for a cachectic patient.
• System requires a special tubing unit.
• Power pack must be recharged weekly.
• Reservoir bag is expensive; it may require changing every 2 to 3 days (depending on the prescribed dosage).
• Needle and tubing must be changed weekly. If irritation develops at the insertion site, the needle may need replacing more frequently.

INFUSAID IMPLANTABLE PUMP

This pump delivers a continuous analgesic infusion from a reservoir chamber to the epidural space. After placing the catheter, the doctor will probably implant the pump subcutaneously in the lower left or right abdominal quadrant or subclavicular area and fill the drug reservoir. A special charging fluid exerts pressure that pumps the drug out through the catheter. The drug reservoir must be refilled every 2 weeks (by injection through the skin into the port) and kept filled at all times with the analgesic (or a replacement fluid, such as normal saline solution). A side port allows intermittent bolus analgesic injections.

Infusaid Implantable Pump

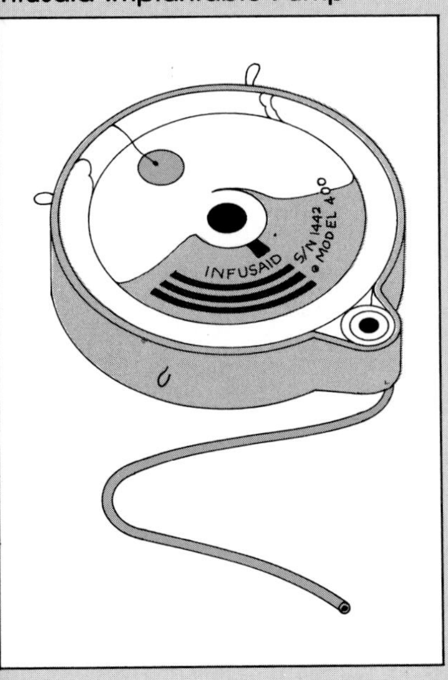

Advantages
• Eliminates the need for an exteriorized central venous catheter and repeated venipuncture
• Maintains continuous analgesic delivery to epidural space
• Allows repeated access for long-term and continuous drug infusion
• Eliminates the need for dressing changes, since none of the equipment is external
• Reduces the risk of infection because the entire system is internal
• Can be used at home
• Doesn't require batteries

Disadvantages
• Insertion requires a surgical procedure.
• Morphine, as well as other drugs, must be specially prepared without preservatives.
• Drug chamber must be refilled every 2 weeks by doctor or specially trained nurse.
• Drug chamber must not be allowed to run dry.
• Between treatments, drug chamber may be filled with normal saline solution.
• Flow rate is dependent on concentration of drug in pump reservoir. Flow rate also varies with body temperature and altitude changes.
• Patient may develop drug tolerance rapidly.

INFUSAID PORT-A-CATH

Similar to the Infusaid Implantable Pump, this implantable system permits intermittent or continuous drug infusion via the I.V. route. (Drugs are delivered by injection through the skin.) However, unlike the Implantable Pump, the Port-a-Cath requires an I.V. set and external I.V. pump to deliver a continuous infusion.

Advantages
• Eliminates the need for an exteriorized central venous catheter, reducing the risk of infection
• Eliminates the need for repeated venipuncture
• Can be used to withdraw blood

Disadvantages
• Port-a-Cath must be flushed regularly with heparinized solution to prevent clotting.
• Patient may develop infection or inflammation around the injection site.
• Catheter may become blocked from a kink in the tubing, occlusion by an intraluminal thrombus, or growth of a fibrin sheath.
• Catheter's distal end may become lodged against the blood vessel wall, right atrium, or peritoneum as the patient moves.

ABBOTT PATIENT-CONTROLLED ANALGESIA (PCA) SYSTEM

This system consists of a portable, computerized pump with a chamber housing a prefilled syringe. The pump delivers the drug through an I.V. catheter. To

CONTINUED ON PAGE 104

SPECIAL INFUSION SYSTEMS CONTINUED

COMPARING A FEW INFUSION SYSTEMS CONTINUED

relieve pain, the patient presses a button at the end of a cord attached to the pump. The syringe releases a small drug dose predetermined by the doctor, providing almost immediate pain relief. The doctor also programs the pump to limit the total drug dosage the patient can administer over a period of time.

Advantages

• Allows the patient to give himself small, intermittent drug doses
• Provides quick and consistent pain relief
• Useful for postoperative pain
• May give the patient a sense of control over pain so he's less anxious and requires less medication
• Has built-in safeguards that prevent unauthorized tampering and overdosing
• Eliminates the need for repeated injections

Disadvantage

• System is less portable than some other systems.

Abbott PCA System

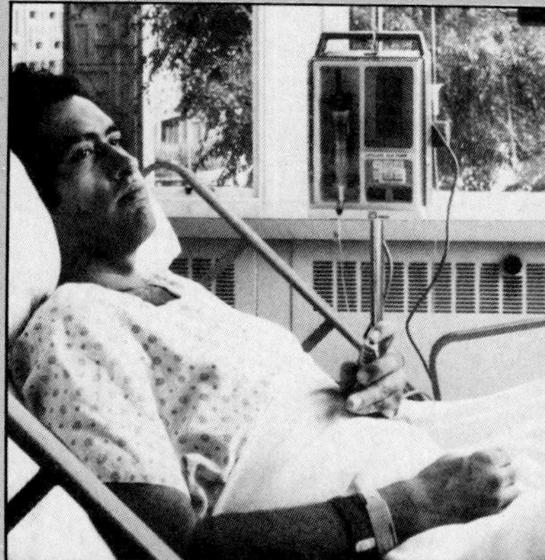

CONTROLLING PAIN WITH EPIDURAL ANALGESIA

Epidural analgesia involves continuous or intermittent administration of a local anesthetic such as bupivacaine hydrochloride (Marcaine) or a narcotic analgesic such as morphine into the epidural space surrounding the spinal cord, as shown in the illustration on page 97. The procedure is currently being used to relieve postoperative, labor, and chronic cancer pain (especially pain associated with sacral and pelvic tumors that have invaded nerves or bone) after more conservative measures become ineffective.

Narcotic analgesics. Administered epidurally, narcotics bind to opiate receptors in the dorsal horn. As a result, they selectively block pain impulses at the spinal cord, causing fewer systemic adverse effects than those caused by other routes. Although narcotics delivered epidurally are absorbed into cerebrospinal fluid (CSF) and the bloodstream, peak drug concentrations are greater in CSF than in blood—and remain significantly higher for several hours. Therefore, the narcotic's effects on the brain stem are minimized, and some patients experience fewer of such adverse effects as sedation, respiratory depression, and nausea.

Nevertheless, adverse narcotic effects are still a risk after epidural administration, so monitor the patient closely. Respiratory depression may occur up to 24 hours after epidural narcotic infusion. An opiate-naive patient (one with no narcotics in his system before the infusion) is at greatest risk.

Anesthetics. Given epidurally, a local anesthetic blocks small-diameter sensory and autonomic nerve fibers more than larger-diameter motor fibers. Temperature impulses are also carried by these small nerve fibers. As a result, the patient feels numbness, decreased temperature sensation, and pain relief distal to the catheter's placement in the spinal cord. For example, if the catheter's placed in your patient's spinal cord at T12 (as in the illustration on page 97), he will experience pain relief beginning from about his waist down.

Because drug effects peak 20 minutes after the infusion, monitor the patient's vital signs 10 to 30 minutes after giving the drug or starting the infusion. If his orthostatic vital signs are normal 30 minutes after beginning the infusion, permit him to walk (if he's able)—but *with assistance only*.

Risks. Epidural infusions can cause serious complications, so they should never be ordered without first considering other alternatives. For example, the catheter could erode into a blood vessel, causing the drug to have systemic effects. If the drug's a narcotic, for example, you'd see such narcotic I.V. effects as sedation. With a local anesthetic, you'd see cardiovascular and cerebrovascular effects such as dysrhythmias, confusion, and possibly seizures. If you suspect drug infusion into the bloodstream, notify the doctor at once and prepare to stop the infusion (if necessary) and assist with catheter repositioning.

For more on possible problems associated with epidural infusions, see the following chart.

MANAGING AN EPIDURAL INFUSION SYSTEM

Epidural analgesia may be administered either intermittently or continuously through an epidural catheter inserted by the doctor, using a technique similar to lumbar puncture. (For continuous infusion, connect the catheter to an infusion pump.) Dosages and intervals are predetermined by an anesthesiologist or neurologist who is solely responsible for adjusting the dosage schedule.

Note: If your patient requires additional analgesic doses, he may receive smaller doses than those normally ordered for a patient who isn't receiving epidural analgesia.

Only specially trained personnel should manage epidural infusion systems, following hospital policy. If you've been specially trained, follow these recommended guidelines:

- Use aseptic technique to prevent catheter-related sepsis.
- Don't try to compensate for infusion lapses by increasing the flow rate.

Throughout the epidural infusion process, stay alert to a number of possible complications. The most serious is respiratory depression. Also monitor the patient for decreased analgesia; this could indicate a break or kink in the catheter or catheter malpositioning.

- If your patient's receiving an anesthetic, regularly assess his bowel and bladder function and lower extremity strength. Also monitor him for hypotension.

Read the chart that follows to familiarize yourself with some potential hazards, and learn what precautions you can take to prevent them. If a problem occurs, follow hospital policy for discontinuing the epidural infusion and immediately notify the doctor.

Epidural catheter placement

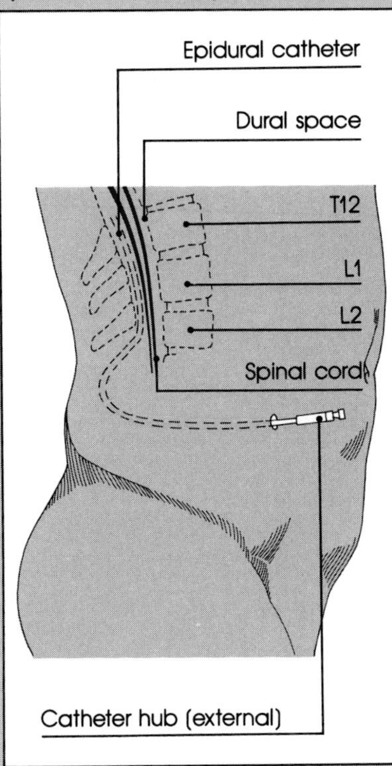

WITH ANESTHETIC OR NARCOTIC USE

PROBLEM

Respiratory depression from subarachnoid medication injection caused by erosion of the catheter into the subarachnoid space. Respiratory depression may also result directly from the drug's effects: an anesthetic depresses respiration by blocking phrenic nerves; a narcotic analgesic depresses the brain's respiratory center.

Signs and symptoms
- Decreased respiratory rate
- Possible hypotension
- Respiratory paralysis

Precautions
- Raise the head of the bed while giving the infusion. Avoid positioning the patient flat because this permits the drug to ascend, which increases the risk of respiratory depression.
- Monitor the patient's vital signs and sensory and motor functions hourly. Establish an I.V. line, and keep naloxone handy to reverse narcotic-induced respiratory depression. Also have a ventilation mask and bag handy.

Interventions
- Assist the doctor with catheter repositioning, if necessary.
- Reduce the drug dosage, if necessary.
- Prepare to initiate supportive measures such as oxygen administration, endotracheal intubation, and ventilatory assistance.

PROBLEM

Spinal headache from puncture of the dura, causing CSF leakage from the spinal cord

Signs and symptoms
- Usually develops 24 hours after epidural catheter insertion
- Produced or exacerbated when the patient sits up

Precaution
- Don't place the patient in upright position for 24 hours after catheter insertion. You may, however, elevate head of bed.

Interventions
- Stop drug infusion.
- Give replacement fluids.

PROBLEM

Infection from poor sterile technique or systemic bacteremia

Signs and symptoms
- Swelling or redness at the insertion site
- Elevated temperature and pulse
- Decreasing sensory and motor function in legs
- Signs of meningitis such as ele-

CONTINUED ON PAGE 106

SPECIAL INFUSION SYSTEMS CONTINUED

MANAGING AN EPIDURAL INFUSION SYSTEM CONTINUED

vated temperature, nuchal rigidity, and changes in mental status

Precautions

- Use aseptic technique to prevent catheter-related infection. (Check hospital policy for epidural catheter care.)
- Use occlusive dressings at the insertion site.

Interventions

- Stop the infusion, and notify the doctor immediately.
- Administer antibiotics, as ordered.
- Monitor the patient's neurologic status closely.
- Use alternative pain-control methods.

PROBLEM

Reversible paraparesis from mistaken infusion of antibiotics, vasopressors, or other drugs with preservatives into the epidural infusion line, causing spinal cord damage

Signs and symptoms

- Paralysis or weakness distal to the catheter insertion site
- Decreased sensation in the legs

Precautions

- Don't allow the patient to walk without assistance.
- Avoid using alcohol wipes to clean the injection ports.
- Secure the catheter lines and dressings to prevent dislodgment.
- Frequently assess the patient's legs for motor strength and sensation.

Interventions

- Stop the drug infusion into the epidural catheter, and notify the doctor immediately.

PROBLEM

Urinary retention. An anesthetic (especially when delivered to the lumbar or sacral region) blocks autonomic innervation of the bladder. A narcotic analgesic (in large doses) inhibits the micturition reflex by direct effect on spinal cord

Signs and symptoms

- Decreased urinary output
- Urinary retention

Precautions

- Maintain fluid intake and output records.
- Assess the patient for bladder distention.

Interventions

- Insert an indwelling (Foley) catheter, as ordered.
- Monitor patient's urine output.

WITH ANESTHETIC USE ONLY

PROBLEM

Hypotension following sympathetic blockade from decreased blood vessel tone

Signs and symptoms

- Hypotension
- Confusion

Precaution

- Monitor the patient's vital signs, especially blood pressure, hourly.

Interventions

- Stop drug and notify doctor. Prepare to give respiratory support.
- Place the patient in a supine position, and elevate his legs.
- Perform passive range-of-motion exercises on his legs.
- Increase the I.V. flow rate, and give sympathomimetic drugs, as ordered.

PROBLEM

Injuries from falls, possibly caused by blockage of motor fibers (particularly in the legs) from high drug concentrations

Signs and symptoms

- Unsteady gait
- Weakness
- Paralysis

Precaution

- Assess the patient's motor strength and sensation regularly. If he can ambulate, provide assistance.

Interventions

- Provide care appropriate to the injury.
- Notify the doctor, and document the incident.

PROBLEM

Systemic toxicity from inadvertent intravascular injection caused by catheter erosion into a blood vessel

Signs and symptoms

- Tingling sensation around the mouth or lips
- Tinnitus
- Tremulousness, shaking, seizures
- Light-headedness
- Confusion, sedation
- Cardiac dysrhythmias

Precautions

- Ask the patient if he's experiencing numbness of his tongue or lips, metallic taste, tinnitus, or vertigo. If he has any of these signs or symptoms of early toxicity, stop the infusion immediately and notify the doctor.
- Observe the patient carefully for convulsions and cardiovascular collapse.

Interventions

- Stop drug and notify doctor.
- Initiate supportive measures to prevent hypoxia and convulsions.
- Administer oxygen (by mask) and diazepam, as ordered.

PEDIATRICS

PRIMARY CONCERNS
ASSESSMENT
INTERVENTION

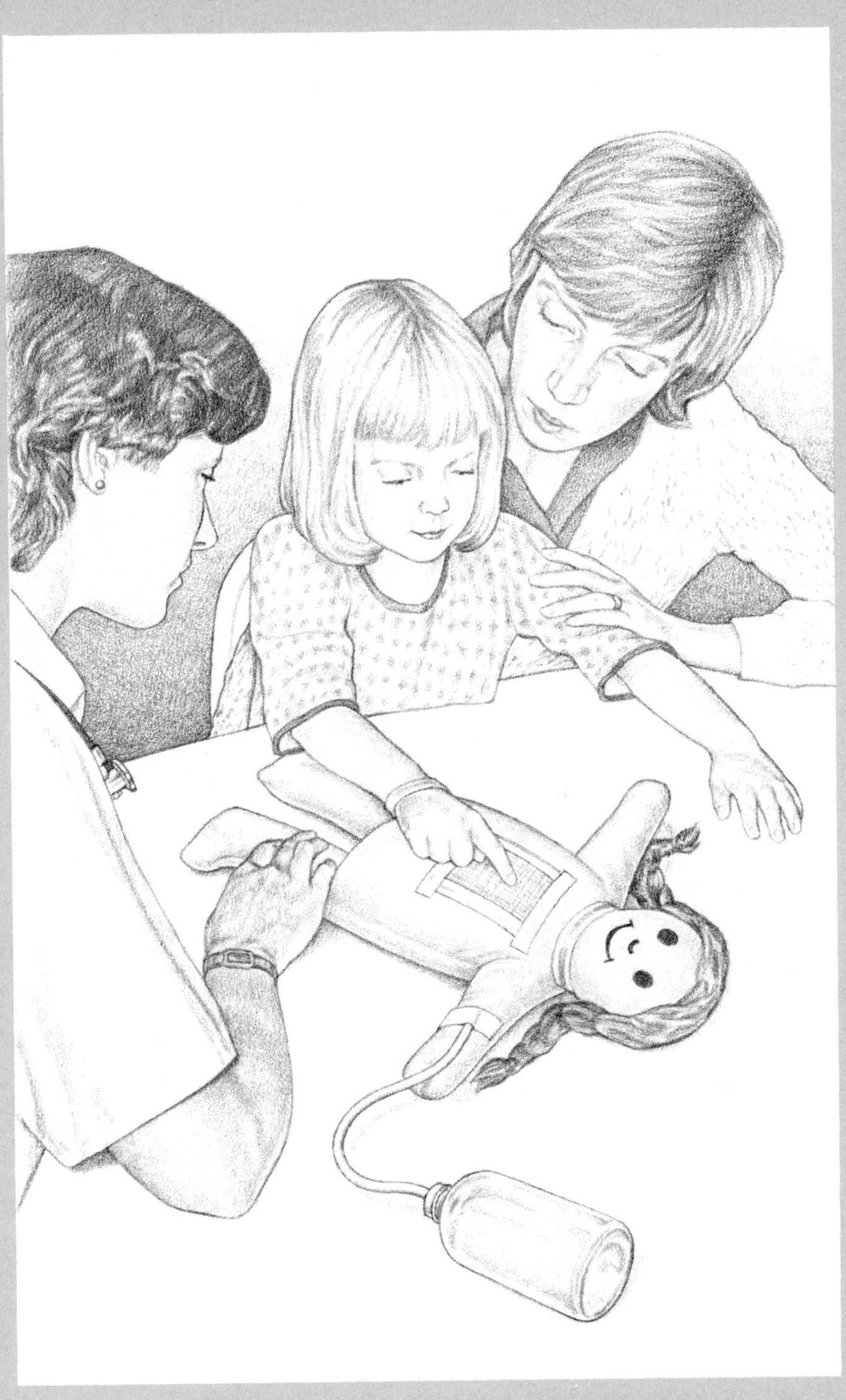

PRIMARY CONCERNS

CHILDREN AND PAIN: A SPECIAL CHALLENGE

Eleven-year-old Lucy Oliver recently completed her first round of chemotherapy for ovarian cancer. Far advanced, the cancer has invaded the spinal nerves and spinal cord, obstructed a ureter, and compressed the bowel.

Chemotherapy was particularly difficult for Lucy, who suffered continual nausea, vomiting, and diarrhea. To complicate matters, the antiemetic given to control her symptoms caused a frightening dystonic drug reaction. From Lucy's viewpoint, medical interventions only added to her problems.

But despite her history and the advanced stage of her cancer, Lucy now adamantly refuses to admit that she has any pain or discomfort. In response to your questions, she consistently denies hurting—and nothing in your assessment findings contradicts her assertions.

Perplexed, you decide to ask her to rate any pain she feels on a scale of 1 to 10. Lucy then surprises you with this reply: "If I say it's a 1, can I go home?"

Afterward, you observe her even more closely. Only then do you realize that, while her behavior appears normal when she's with others, she literally doubles over with pain when she thinks she's alone. Knowing her history, you're not surprised—but you *are* surprised at how effectively the child has disguised her pain.

Although such behavior is unusual among adults, it's not uncommon among children. For a child like Lucy, the hospital represents painful or unpleasant procedures. Unlike an adult, she has difficulty appreciating the relationship between a painful treatment—even an analgesic injection—and future pain relief. From her point of view, admitting to pain simply stands in the way of returning home.

Managing the pain of a child like Lucy presents a unique challenge to your nursing skills. To meet it, you must first recognize that a child views pain, hospitalization—and you—differently than an adult does. You may also need to shed some misconceptions that interfere with effective assessment and intervention. On the next few pages, we'll discredit some widely held myths about children and pain. Then, we'll discuss the assessment techniques and nursing interventions that work best with children.

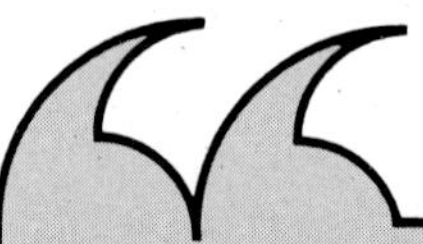

"Because a child isn't a miniature adult, we can't always use adult criteria to assess his pain. But like an adult, he has the right to be pain-free. As nurses, we must make sure he gets the relief he needs, despite the problems he has understanding what he's feeling and telling us about it."

Jo Eland, RN, PhD
Assistant Professor of Nursing
College of Nursing
University of Iowa
Iowa City

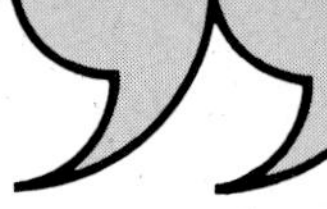

DISPELLING MYTHS ABOUT CHILDREN IN PAIN

Do you believe that children tol erate pain better than adults? O that a child will almost always te you when he hurts? If so, yo share some common misconcep tions about children and pain tha probably limit your ability to in tervene effectively. Consider th following eight myths and hov they can influence pediatric pai management.

MYTH #1

Because their nervous system are immature, children don't fee pain as intensely as adults do.

Because nerves aren't com pletely myelinated at birth health-care professionals once thought that infants can't fee pain with the same intensity tha adults feel it. This myth has per sisted despite compelling com mon-sense evidence to the contrary; an alert newborn un dergoing circumcision withou anesthesia, for example, leaves little doubt about his ability to fee pain (although some people mis interpret his cries as a protest against restraint rather than pain).

We now know that myelination (which progresses rapidly after birth) isn't necessary for pain transmission. Children not only feel pain in much the same way that adults do, some research suggests that they're even more sensitive and that pain thresholds increase with age.

MYTH #2

If a child's active, he can't be feeling much pain.

Too often, we evaluate a child's pain response in adult terms. When we observe, for example, that a child becomes ambulatory more quickly than an adult who's undergone the same surgical procedure, we may be tempted to conclude that the child has recovered more quickly and that he's feeling less pain. But for a child, activity may be a coping technique that helps him deal with pain and anxiety. For example, many mothers can tell you that their toddlers become more—not less—active when suffering from such a painful condition as an acute ear infection.

A hospitalized child may have additional incentive for early ambulation: he may associate his hospital bed with such painful or unpleasant procedures as injections, venipuncture, and suctioning. To avoid these procedures, the child may try to escape from his room as often as possible. Many children up to age 14 believe that, if they physically remove themselves from a place they associate with a painful event, the painful event won't recur. In fact, the credo of many experienced hospitalized children seems to be "Keep moving and stay out of your room."

MYTH #3

A child can't tell you where he hurts.

Certainly, a child isn't likely to give a detailed, clinical account of the location and quality of his pain. But he can effectively communicate what he's feeling in terms appropriate to his age and personal experiences. For example, one child recovering from surgery for heel cord lengthening described his leg as feeling "like a lemon." Although this response at first seems inappropriate, his meaning becomes clear when he goes on to say, "You know how, when you have a lemon drop in your cheek for a long time and then take it away, your cheek feels shriveled? Well, that's how my leg feels." Another child may describe knee pain as "having a headache in my knee," because headache is one of the few painful experiences he's familiar with.

Keep in mind that pain is a difficult concept for a child to learn, largely because pain is a subjective and variable experience. Ischemic muscle pain, headache, indigestion, and venipuncture cause distinctly different sensations, and the child may not associate them all with the word *pain*. As a matter of fact, a child as old as age 10 may not even know what the word *pain* means. In contrast, one study showed that adults use more than 140 words to describe all the dimensions of pain.

A young child learns pain concepts more easily when the pain is associated with an objective consequence; for example, when he associates abdominal pain with vomiting. Pain without such an easily identifiable consequence—headache pain, for example—may be more difficult for him to conceptualize.

Don't assume that a child can't tell you about his pain simply because he hasn't learned an adult's pain vocabulary. By using appropriate assessment tools, you can help even very young children describe their pain to you—with remarkable clarity. We'll discuss assessment guidelines beginning on page 111.

MYTH #4

A child always accurately describes his own pain.

When your patient's an adult, you consider him to be the best judge of his own pain. But with a child, following this usually reliable rule of thumb is sometimes a mistake. Why? For several reasons. First, although even a young child is capable of telling you where he hurts, he may refuse to do so because he fears the consequence: an analgesic injection, which he associates with *more* pain, not pain relief. Or he may believe that he'll be discharged sooner if he denies having pain.

Another reason is that a child may not recognize pain until after it's gone. When pain onset is gradual, as in some types of cancer, the child may learn to cope with it, unconsciously accepting it as a normal part of life. Such was the case with Loren, a silent, withdrawn 13-year-old with widespread Ewing's sarcoma. Although Loren's disease was far advanced, he repeatedly denied feeling pain. But based on knowledge of the child's disease and its metastasis, his nurses concluded that Loren *must be* in pain despite his denials and asked the doctor to order round-the-clock analgesics. After administering analgesics for 36 hours, the nurses saw a dramatic change in Loren—no longer quiet and withdrawn, he behaved like a normal, outgoing teenager. When asked again about his pain, Loren replied, "I think I had been hurting for so long that I forgot what it was like *not* to hurt."

As Loren's story illustrates, this myth is particularly insidious because it encourages us to ignore a child's pain when he doesn't admit having it. As a result, he's deprived of the pain relief he may desperately need.

CONTINUED ON PAGE 110

PRIMARY CONCERNS CONTINUED

DISPELLING MYTHS ABOUT CHILDREN IN PAIN CONTINUED

MYTH #5

Narcotic analgesics are dangerous for children because of the danger of addiction.

Elsewhere in this book, we've discussed how the fear of causing narcotic addiction may prevent health-care professionals from providing effective pain relief for adults in severe pain. When the patients are children, this fear is even more exaggerated. Yet, as with adults, the risk of addiction in children is small—and virtually nonexistent when the drugs are given only for short-term pain relief; for example, following surgery.

As with any drug, you must weigh potential risks against expected benefits. A child who's pain-free following surgery can cooperate with coughing, deep breathing, and early ambulation.

When only narcotics can control the severe pain of a terminal illness, the question of addiction becomes irrelevant. Under these circumstances, pain relief may be all you can offer the child. Nevertheless, fear of causing addiction can lead health-care professionals to give ineffective dosages far below recommended levels. No nurse would withhold insulin from a diabetic child who needs it, even though he may need the drug for the rest of his life. To a health-care professional, intractable, terminal pain should be as unacceptable as hyperglycemia.

MYTH #6

Narcotic analgesics are likely to cause dangerous respiratory depression in children.

Again, this fear has been exaggerated beyond the actual risk. Of course, respiratory depression is a possible adverse effect of narcotics; you'd assess any patient for neurologic and respiratory conditions that contraindicate narcotic administration. But in the absence of contraindications, the risk of respiratory depression is small. Don't hesitate to give a narcotic, as ordered, when your assessment findings reveal no contraindications.

MYTH #7

The best way to give analgesics is by injection.

To many children, the pain associated with an injection is the worst pain they've ever had. Though an adult recognizes the relationship between an analgesic injection and pain relief, a child simply associates the injection with more pain. Consider the results of one survey. Out of 186 hospitalized children between ages 4 and 10 who were asked, "Of all the things that have ever hurt you, what was the worst?", 62% answered, "Shot or needle." Among them were six children who'd undergone 25 or more surgical procedures.

A child's fear of an injection—coupled with our reluctance to inflict pain on a child—clearly suggests that injection (particularly by the painful I.M. route) is *not* the best way to give analgesics to children. Yet many health-care professionals continue to believe that no effective alternatives exist.

As we'll discuss in the section beginning on page 116, you can give many powerful analgesics by oral, rectal, or I.V. routes. And when I.M. injections are unavoidable, you can deaden the pain with topical anesthetics such as Frigiderm.

MYTH #8

Parents are the best judges of their child's pain.

Although parents know their own child better than anyone, they're at a disadvantage when he's hospitalized. They may misjudge the child's pain because:

- they've never seen the child in so much pain before and don't know what behavior to expect under the circumstances.
- they themselves are upset by the hospital experience.
- they believe that nurses and other staff members, who care for sick children every day, are better judges of the child's condition. As one mother said, "A nurse would know if my child hurt. She wouldn't let him lie there and suffer."

In general, parents are a pediatric nurse's best allies. But although their observations and suggestions are often invaluable, you must rely heavily on your own assessment skills to evaluate a child's pain and his response to treatment.

ASSESSMENT

CHILDREN IN PAIN: A SPECIAL CHALLENGE

On page 109, we introduced Loren, a 13-year-old patient who said, "I think I'd been hurting for so long that I forgot what it was like *not* to hurt."

His story illustrates a problem you may encounter when assessing a child's pain: if his pain evolved slowly, he may have become so accustomed to it that it seems normal.

The difficulty some children have in recognizing their own pain is only one of many challenges you face. You'll also be confronted with the denial of pain by those children who fear the treatment—most likely, an analgesic injection—more than the pain. And you'll have to find ways of communicating with children who don't know the names of their body parts and who aren't even sure what the word *pain* means.

Throughout the following pages, we'll discuss the special considerations you should keep in mind when assessing a child for pain. You'll learn ways of recognizing pain, even in children who, like Loren, deny hurting. You'll also see how different stages of cognitive development can affect a child's responses to and reports of pain. In addition, we'll show you how to talk to children about their pain and give you some specific tools to help you assess pain in your pediatric patients.

WHAT AFFECTS A CHILD'S PAIN RESPONSE?

Pain is subjective and personal. No two people experience it in the same way, at the same intensity, or for the same reasons—and this is as true for children as for adults. Before assessing a child for pain, consider the following variables that can affect his perception of pain and his responses to it.

Prior pain experience. If your pediatric patient's had pain previously, beware of making assumptions about how it will affect his response to current or anticipated pain. If you expect him to be especially apprehensive and fearful, he could surprise you. Many children with long histories of illness, accidents, and hospitalizations become stoic in the face of pain. On the other hand, some children with no prior pain history—not counting the usual childhood bumps and scrapes—become terrified when they have significant pain for the first time.

To assess the effect of prior experience, ask your pediatric patient if he's ever been in the hospital before. Does he remember ever feeling really sick or hurt? Ask him to relate any painful experiences he may have had.

Watch the child as he answers your questions. Does he appear tense and anxious or matter-of-fact? His attitude toward these past experiences may give you important clues about how he will respond to pain now. You might also ask him what he expects to happen and then explain what really will happen to him.

Note: Some children refuse to talk in stressful situations. Try to find nonverbal ways to communicate; for example, through pictures.

Interviewing parents can also help you anticipate your pediatric patient's response to pain, especially if the child is very young or is unable or unwilling to talk to you. The child may be too young to remember past painful experiences, or he may have blocked those experiences from conscious memory. The child's medical history should give you a good starting point for your questions.

Advance preparation. A child who knows in advance what to expect from a medical procedure is less likely to respond with the fear, anger, and frustration that can intensify pain. By warning the child that a procedure is going to hurt (it even helps to tell him how much and for how long), you give him the opportunity to rehearse the experience and bring all his coping mechanisms into full play. Although

CONTINUED ON PAGE 112

Preoperative preparation

Using a doll as a teaching aid, you can help prepare a child to handle the pain and stress of a painful procedure, such as heart surgery.

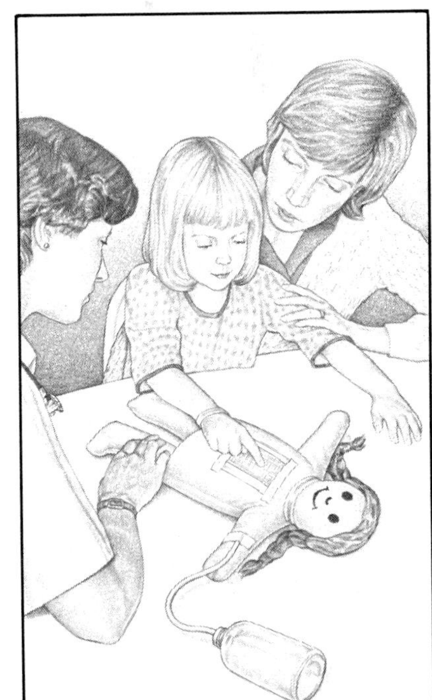

ASSESSMENT CONTINUED

WHAT AFFECTS A CHILD'S PAIN RESPONSE? CONTINUED

it may be easier for *you* to surprise your patient with a painful procedure (you won't have to listen to his crying or restrain his thrashing arms and legs), such a tactic makes the experience worse for the child. And in the long run, you'll probably only lose his trust.

Birth order. Some scientists have suggested that birth order can affect a child's response to pain. Firstborn and only children seem to be more likely than later-born children to become anxious when anticipating pain. After all, later-born children have the advantage of observing their older brothers or sisters and rehearsing pain experiences in play. So, when preparing your patient for a painful procedure or determining just how much pain a crying child is really feeling, find out his birth order. Then anticipate that a firstborn may require more comforting.

Sex differences. Boys feel pain just as much as girls do. Don't encourage a boy to behave like a little man; such unrealistic expectations only make the child feel inadequate if he finds he can't bear up stoically under pain. Instead, encourage all your pediatric patients to express their feelings in ways that come naturally to them—regardless of sex.

Age. Because of developmental changes, children respond to pain differently at different ages. A toddler may scream for his mommy; fear of separation is a big factor in his pain. An adolescent may just grit his teeth; he fears loss of the autonomy and control he's been struggling so hard to attain. At right, we'll discuss developmental stages in more detail and give you an idea of what to expect from children in different age-groups.

CONSIDERING A CHILD'S DEVELOPMENTAL STAGE

A child's age bears directly on his responses to pain and on his ability to tell you about it. The following points, based on Piaget's stages of cognitive development, should help you better understand a child's behavior and assess his pain.

• *Preschool age (age 18 months to 5 years).* Most younger preschoolers don't understand everything that's happening to them during a hospital stay. Because their thinking is egocentric, they expect you to know what they know and to automatically understand what they are feeling. They may be unable to separate you from the pain and consider you to be the cause of it.

Preschoolers employ what psychologists call *precausal* or *magical* reasoning: making cause-and-effect associations between events that are connected only in time. For example, if a child hurts his foot immediately after being scolded by his mother, he may believe that the injury is a punishment for bad behavior. A preschooler may also fantasize that common hospital equipment, such as a respirator or an I.V. pump, is a terrible monster trying to hurt him.

A preschooler's biggest fear is separation from his parents. For a child this age, separation is as final and devastating as death is to an adult. This child needs close contact with his parents and derives comfort from such transitional objects as a stuffed toy or a so-called security blanket.

• *School-age (age 5 to 11).* The thinking of school-age children is more flexible than that of preschoolers. These older children can consider viewpoints other than their own and readily discard notions that are proven incorrect. But they still think largely in concrete terms. Not yet adept at abstract thinking, they relate experiences to physical experience—what they have seen, heard, felt, touched, and tasted. Although more logical than preschoolers, they may still believe that hospitalization is a punishment for some misdeed.

School-age children are problem solvers. They need and demand explanations that you should be ready to give. They're also fascinated with their bodies and will want to understand everything that's being done to them. Just remember to use concrete terms, and be ready to illustrate your answers with drawings and hospital equipment.

"I once had an 8-year-old patient who suffered a spiral leg fracture from a skateboard accident. Knowing that the fracture had to be painful, I repeatedly asked her if she was in pain—using appropriate synonyms like *hurt* and *owie*. She consistently shook her head or said, 'No.' Finally, I got smart and asked a simple, open-ended question: 'How does your leg feel now?' To this she replied, 'Sore.' That's when I realized that, for this child, *sore* meant *pain*. Throughout her hospitalization, *sore* was the only word she ever used for *pain*."

Jo Eland, RN, PhD
Assistant Professor of Nursing
College of Nursing
University of Iowa
Iowa City

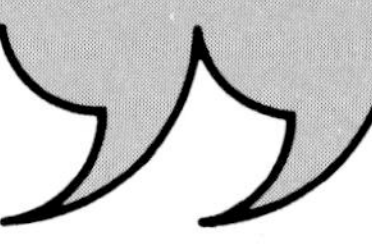

School-age children understand time more fully than preschoolers do. But even though they comprehend what is meant by past, present, and future, they have only a limited memory of past events.

A school-age child may fear mutilation; for example, he may imagine that his throat will be slit during a tonsillectomy.

• *Adolescence (age 11 to 17).* Adolescents are capable of fairly mature reasoning. In fact, their thinking is similar to that of adults. Adolescents value that ability and bristle at simplistic explanations. Be prepared to give as full an explanation of events as your adolescent patients wish. And be sure to give them plenty of time to explain their feelings and beliefs: they need to be listened to.

Typically rebellious, adolescents may balk at rigid rules and inflexible hospital procedures. They need to feel some control over what's happening to them. Pain and the anxiety it creates can make teenagers feel out of control—and as you know, anxiety and stress increase pain. Teenagers also fear mutilation and death.

Allay these fears by explaining procedures and encouraging adolescents to participate in their own care. Because teenagers also derive comfort from the presence of friends and family members (sometimes siblings are more welcome than parents), encourage visitors when appropriate and permit patients to engage in regular interests and hobbies whenever possible.

CRITICAL QUESTIONS

CLUES: ASSESSING A CHILD'S BEHAVIOR

Children express pain eloquently with body language. If your patient is too young to describe his pain verbally, his behavior may be your *only* indication of how he feels.

Behavior that reflects pain varies among children. Some respond by becoming quiet and withdrawn. Others, perhaps attempting to escape pain, become more active. The key is to identify behavior that's unusual for the child you're assessing.

Of course, the child's parents can provide valuable insights. But don't underestimate the value of your nursing instincts and assessment skills. You should listen to what the child says, watch for behavioral changes, monitor his condition for physiologic changes, and know the pathology of his disease or condition.

During your assessment, ask yourself the following questions. Thoroughly document all your observations and findings.

• *Is the child quiet or talkative?* Does he ask to be left alone or ask for company? Does he express his fears and desires? Does he call for his mother or father? Is his behavior around others consistent? Or is he quiet with some people and talkative with others?

• *How does he express himself nonverbally?* A withdrawn child may sleep excessively, assume a fetal position, clutch a favorite toy, hide under the covers, or repeatedly turn away from people. An extroverted child expresses himself by reaching out to others, crying, clinging, and perhaps biting or hitting those around him.

• *How does he describe his pain?* Does he say he's in pain—or deny pain? Can he tell you what hurts? Can he tell you what his pain feels like?

• *Is he eating well?* If not, does he play with the food or push it away? Does he seem reluctant to swallow?

• *What other behavior do you see that might reflect pain?* For example, does he pace, jump on his bed, fidget, or toss and turn? Or does he sit or lie rigidly, walk or stand hunched over, or grind his teeth? Note his facial expressions, too—wincing, grimacing, and a clenched jaw all suggest pain.

ASSESSMENT CONTINUED

GUIDELINES FOR TALKING WITH CHILDREN

In some ways, talking to a child is more challenging than talking to an adult. But conducting an informative interview with a child really isn't difficult, if you keep these special considerations in mind:

- Let the child know you care about him, with your body language as well as your words. Direct eye contact, gentle touching, and inclining your body toward him encourages his trust and confidence.
- Show you're listening and interested in what he has to say. Don't interrupt him or finish his sentences.
- Tailor your vocabulary to the child's age and intellect. Remember, not all children understand the word *pain.* If your patient's very young, words like *hurt, ouch,* and *owie* may mean more to him.
- Ask open-ended questions; this technique helps you avoid putting words in the child's mouth. For example, instead of asking him if his head (or other painful body part) hurts, ask him how his head feels. Then, listen carefully to his answer. Try to find out what words signify pain to him.
- Avoid using big or technical words that the child won't understand. Also, beware of using terms the child could misinterpret. For example, a child might mistakenly believe that *dye* means *die.*
- Avoid words or expressions with negative connotations. For example, a child who's told he'll be "put to sleep" for an operation may think of unwanted animals that are killed in animal shelters. Instead of using terms like *cut, take out,* or *suture,* which could upset a child, try using such neutral words as *fix.*

When interviewing a child, give him every opportunity to express his fears and to ask questions.

- Find ways of explaining unfamiliar concepts in terms the child can understand. Concrete analogies help. In explaining heart procedures, for example, you might describe the heart as a pump and show the child a working model.

USING A NUMBER SCALE

In addition to the Eland Color Tool described at right, a simple number scale can help you assess a child's pain. If he's old enough to understand that 5 is more than 1, he can learn to rate his pain numerically. Use a scale ranging from 0 to 10 or from 0 to 5, depending on the child's mathematical sophistication. On either scale, 0 represents no pain and the largest number the worst pain.

As in using the Eland Color Tool, combine number scales with interviews. Get the child to tell you about the worst pain he's ever experienced. Make that pain the largest number on your scale. Give smaller numbers to smaller hurts.

Important: Be specific with the assignment of each number. A child understands pain better when he can refer to examples rather than an abstract concept.

After you've discussed the degrees of hurt, ask the child to tell you how much he hurts now, using one of the numbers.

THE ELAND COLOR TOOL: ILLUSTRATING PAIN

Designed for use during an interview, the Eland Color Tool lets the child show you what hurts and how much. In addition to its value during assessment, this tool can provide early diagnostic clues to disease.

To use the Eland Color Tool, obtain a set of crayons and body outlines. (Copy the teaching aid at right for use during the interview.) Then, follow these steps.

- Ask the child, "What kinds of things have hurt you before?"
- If he doesn't answer, ask, "Has anyone ever stuck your finger for blood? What did that feel like?"
- After discussing several things that have hurt the child in the past, ask, "Of all the things that have ever hurt you, what was the worst?"
- Give the child eight crayons and ask him, "Of these colors, which is like the thing that hurt you the most?" *Important:* Name the painful incident specifically.
- Place the crayon representing severe pain to one side.
- Ask, "Which color is like a hurt, but not as bad as your worst hurt?" (Again, specifically name the hurt.)
- Place the second crayon next to the one representing severe pain.
- Continue in this way, choosing crayons that represent just a little hurt and no hurt at all.
- Give the four chosen crayons to the child along with the body outlines. You might write the child's name above or below the outline.
- Ask the child to use his crayons to show you on the outline where he hurts a lot, a middle amount, just a little, or not at all.
- Ask, "Is this hurt happening right now, or is it from earlier today? Does it happen all the time or on and off?"
- Remember to include a color key on the tool.
- Document all the child's responses, using his own words.

FOR THE PATIENT

WHERE DO YOU HURT?

Color these pictures to show where you hurt. Use the crayons you and the nurse picked out. When you finish coloring, give the pictures to the nurse.

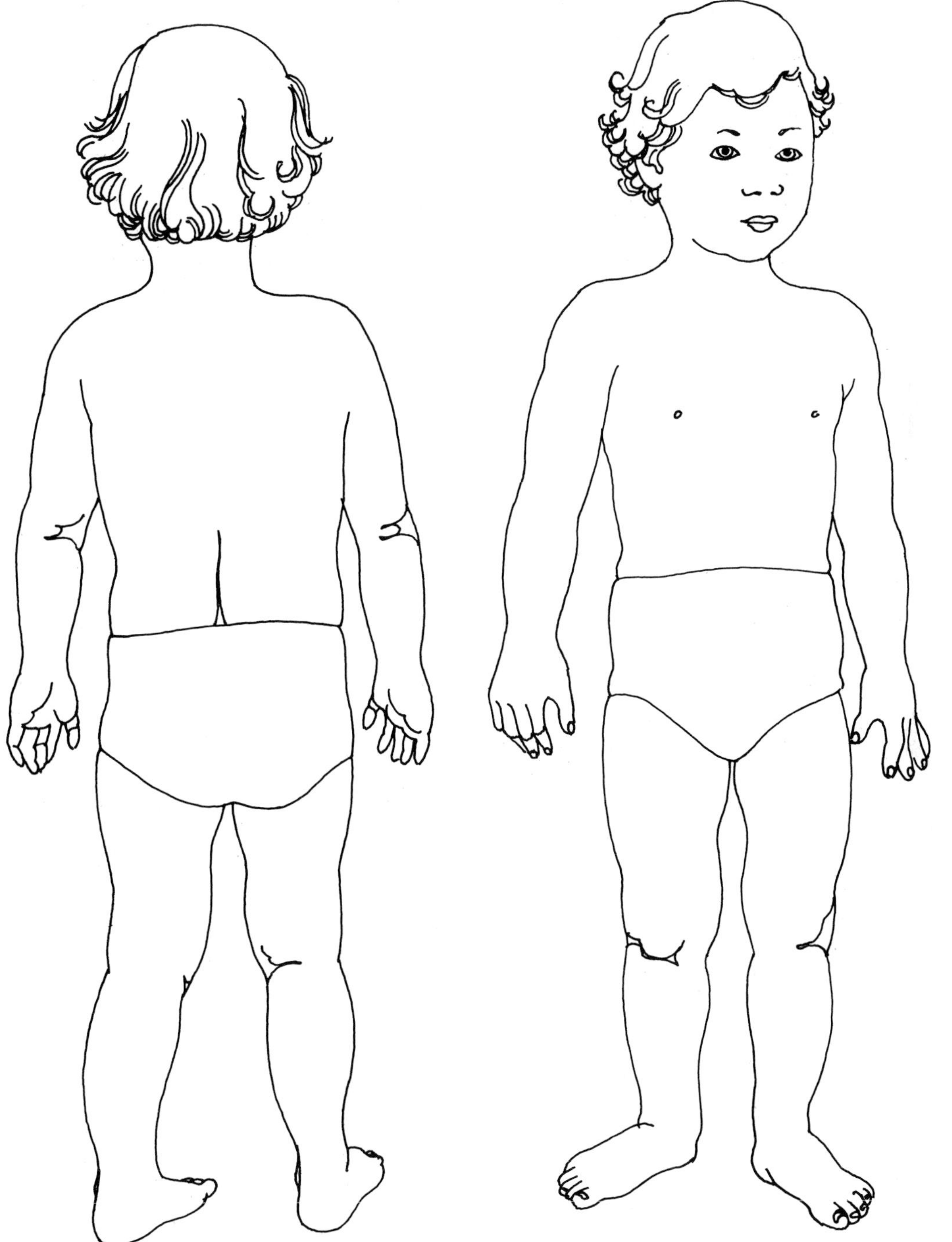

INTERVENTION

CASE IN POINT

A NURSE'S DILEMMA: INFLICTING PAIN TO RELIEVE PAIN

Alison Cole, a talkative and good-natured 5-year-old, is recovering from a nephrectomy. The orientation kit she received from the hospital before admission prepared her well. Before surgery, she told you about the bad cells the doctor planned to remove from her kidney so that her tummy wouldn't hurt anymore. And she showed you where the doctor would make the incision. Unfortunately, no one told Alison about the injections of meperidine hydrochloride (Demerol) the doctor would order after the surgery (35 mg every 3 hours).

Now, a day later, this normally active and fun-loving child is in severe pain. She's also frustrated and angry. The Demerol injection you just administered made her cry. And so far, it hasn't made her pain go away as you said it would. "You're a mean nurse!" she screams at you.

At this moment, you may agree with Alison. You feel guilty about inflicting more pain on a child who's already suffering. No one wants to make a child cry—you were simply trying to relieve her pain. But despite their therapeutic benefits, injections are painful. How can you avoid being a "bad guy" and yet manage Alison's pain effectively?

Before answering that question, let's first mention what you *shouldn't* do. Never allow your guilt and frustration to interfere with your sound nursing judgment. If you do, you may find yourself avoiding subsequent injections or administering as few as possible. The result: an undermedicated child who endures needless pain.

Instead, take steps to make analgesic administration bearable for a child and for yourself. The information below will help.

ADMINISTERING ANALGESICS TO A CHILD

For most children, the pain of an injection seems worse than the underlying pain it's intended to relieve. Unlike an adult, who knows that pain relief will follow, a child can't make a connection between immediate injection pain and future pain relief. From his viewpoint, the injection simply hurts and makes him feel worse.

Of all injection types, I.M. injections are the most painful. Avoid them whenever possible. With proper dosage adjustment, many analgesics are effective in oral, I.V., or rectal forms. For example, morphine and methadone can be given orally; continuous infusions of morphine given with an infusion pump can also keep a child pain-free without subjecting him to repeated I.M. injections. Oxymorphone hydrochloride (Numorphan) is effective in suppository form. If the doctor has ordered an I.M. analgesic and the drug is available in another form, discuss the options with him.

When giving an I.M. injection is unavoidable, minimize the child's fear and discomfort by following these guidelines. (Use them when you use other parenteral routes, too.)

- Explain why you're giving the injection in terms he can understand. For example, you might tell him that the injection will make him feel better but not right away. Explain that the medicine must travel through his body to the hurt part before he'll feel better. To use a guided imagery technique, encourage him to imagine the medicine traveling through his body.
- Be honest with the child. Tell him that the injection will hurt, but emphasize that his cooperation will make it hurt less.
- Give the child as much control as possible. For example, let him choose the arm or buttock to use as the injection site.
- Use a topical anesthetic, such as Frigiderm, to minimize injection pain. Explain that the Frigiderm will make his skin feel cold, so the injection won't hurt as much. To use Frigiderm, cleanse the skin, spray Frigiderm on the site for 3 to 5 seconds, and give the injection. *Note:* Frigiderm doesn't alter pain associated with tissue irritation caused by a drug such as meperidine.
- Help the child to relax by asking him to wiggle his toes or to count.
- Don't ask parents to restrain the child. If necessary, ask a co-worker to help; comfort the child afterward.
- Tell the child that he may cry if he wants. Give him a pillow or a stuffed toy to punch, if he'd like.
- If he wishes, apply a colorful adhesive bandage strip to the site. A bandage makes some younger children feel protected; it also acts as a badge of courage.

I.M. injection sites

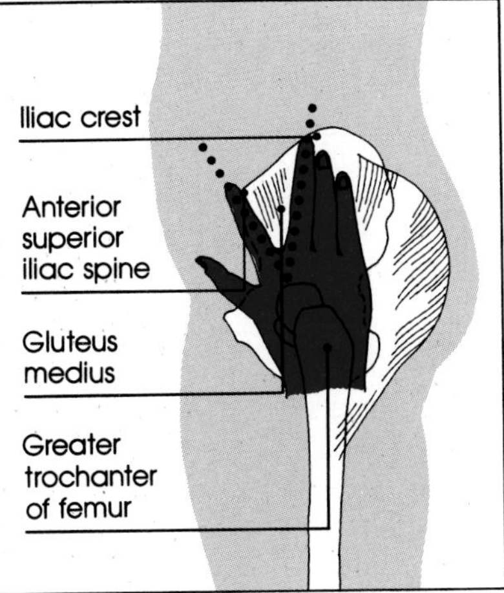

Ventrogluteal
Make this site your first choice when giving an I.M. injection to a child; it's probably the least painful. (Although some authorities discourage ventrogluteal injections for children under age 3, this stance is controversial.) To give an injection, position the child on his back—you needn't turn him to his side. Insert the needle in the area within the dotted lines.

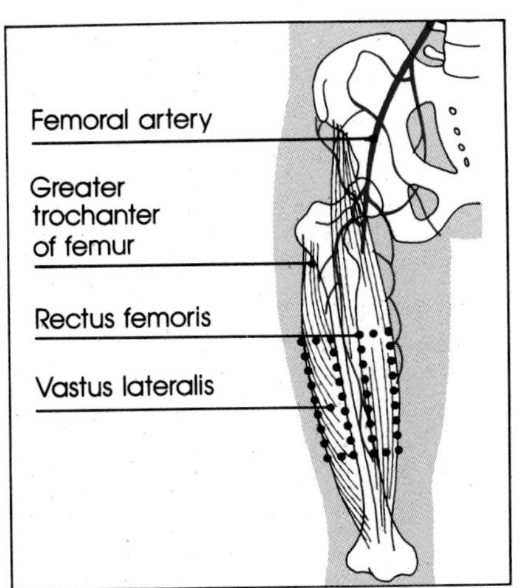

Vastus lateralis and rectus femoris
These sites (indicated above by the rectangular outlines) are alternatives for children of all ages. Because they contain few major vessels and nerves, the risk of injury is minimal. However, these sites are more painful than others.

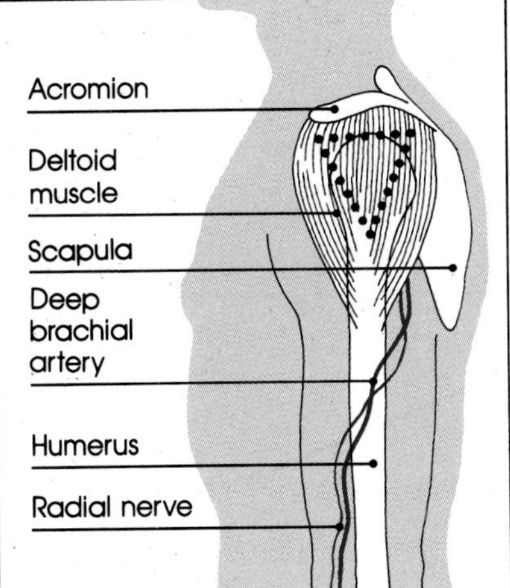

Deltoid
A disadvantage of this site (see the triangular outline above) is that it's near the radial nerve. Also, because the muscle is small, you can give only small drug doses here. But drugs given here may take effect faster than drugs given at other I.M. sites.

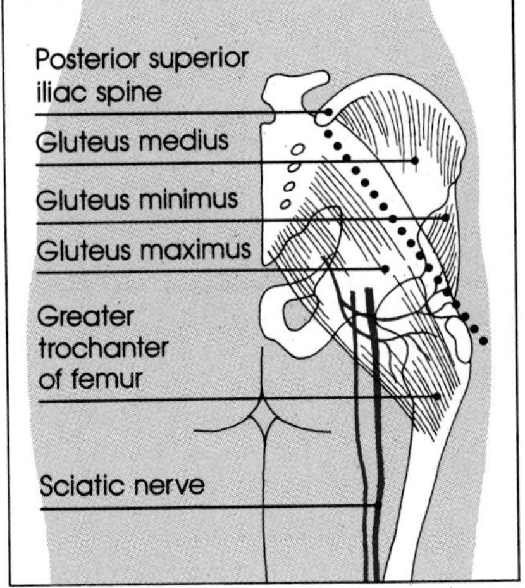

Dorsogluteal
Many authorities don't recommend this site for children under age 3; however, as with the ventrogluteal site, this opinion is controversial. Restrict injections to the area above and outside the dotted line drawn from the posterior superior iliac spine to the greater trochanter of the femur.

GIVING MORPHINE: TWO ALTERNATE ROUTES

In recent years, many children with severe pain have gotten relief from continuous I.V. morphine infusions. The I.V. route eliminates the need for repeated injections, allows rapid onset of action, and produces a steady level of analgesia. Continuous I.V. morphine is the preferred route for patients with:

- intractable vomiting
- severe pain that's unrelieved by oral or intermittent parenteral narcotics
- severe local bruising following subcutaneous or I.M. drug administration.

You can also administer morphine orally. But because of the first-pass effect, oral morphine metabolizes more quickly than I.M. morphine. Expect the doctor to order oral doses that are significantly higher than I.M. doses; dosage intervals will also be shorter.

Another disadvantage of oral morphine is its unpleasant taste. Make it more palatable by using an oral syringe to deposit the drug at the back of the child's tongue to avoid the most sensitive taste buds. If the child's old enough, allow him to administer the morphine himself.

Note: Oral morphine often causes nausea and vomiting. As ordered, give an oral antiemetic about 1 hour before giving oral morphine.

Special Note:

Use extreme caution before giving aspirin to a child under age 13. In children, the drug has been associated with development of Reye's syndrome, a potentially fatal encephalopathy.

INTERVENTION CONTINUED

THERAPEUTIC PLAY: NOT JUST GAMES

For a child, playing is a way to sort out confusing experiences and feelings. Through play, he can better understand information about a painful procedure and express any fears, fantasies, and conflicts the procedure arouses.

Use therapeutic play to prepare a child for a painful experience—think of it as a sort of rehearsal. Obtain a doll, and gather other props you'll need; for example, syringes, sutures, or I.V. tubing. Then, using the doll, perform the procedure while the child watches. Your actions reinforce and clarify your verbal explanation. If the child's old enough, allow him to do the procedure himself. Encourage him to ask questions and express fears.

By becoming familiar with the equipment, this play rehearsal may reduce the child's fear of the unknown. For an older child, the rehearsal is also a chance for him to pretend he's a doctor or nurse.

Using play to prepare a child for I.V. therapy

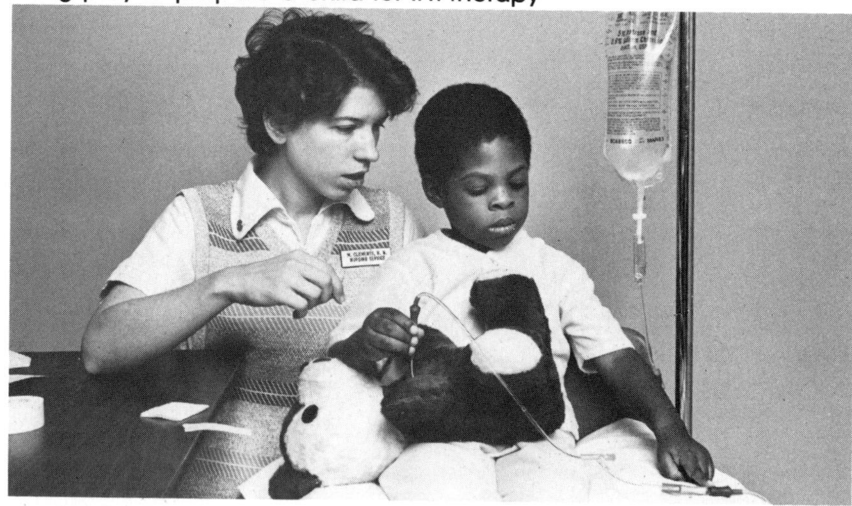

In the process, he may begin to understand that your intent is to help him get better, not to inflict more pain.

Therapeutic play is equally valuable *after* the painful procedure, because it can help the child assimilate the experience and resolve anger and resentment he may feel. Many adults cope with an unpleasant experience by talking about it. But children, who are less articulate, may cope better through play.

Note: Observing a child at play can give you insight into how well he understands your explanations and can help you avoid misunderstandings in the future.

HELPING A CHILD COPE

Nonpharmacologic pain interventions are limited only by your imagination. You can adapt almost any cognitive strategy to help a child cope with pain.

Distraction techniques, for example, work well with children. Have the child choose a song or jingle and tell him to sing it silently or aloud. While he's singing, urge him to keep time by tapping a finger or his foot, nodding his head, or slapping his thigh. Tell the child to sing faster if his pain worsens and to slow down as his pain subsides. Having him listen to tapes through a headset or watch television or a videotape is also an effective distraction technique.

Storytelling is another cognitive strategy well suited to a child; it incorporates elements of distraction and imagery. Or, you can show the child a series of pictures and ask him to tell a story about each one. Encourage him to provide as many details as possible.

When the hurt is gone. Always find a way to let a child know when a painful procedure is over. Your signal reduces his anxiety and helps him to relax. For example, if the child was lying down during the procedure, sit him up as soon as it's complete. If he's very young, pick him up and cuddle him, or show him a toy or give him a snack. If the child is older, take him out of the room to let him know that the painful experience is over.

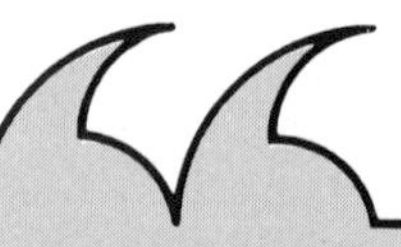

"When you talk to a child, don't use the word *shot* when you mean *injection.* I've cared for children who immediately imagined being shot with a gun. Getting an injection is upsetting enough for a child—to avoid adding to his anxiety, choose your words carefully."

Barbara McVan, RN
Springhouse, Pa.

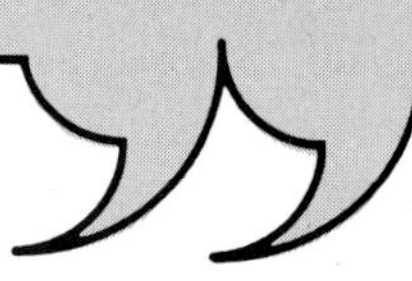

APPENDIX

PAIN-CONTROL CENTERS

If your patient with chronic, intractable pain asks about other treatment options, you may want to refer him to a pain-control or stress center. The pain centers listed below are among the most well established in the United States.

If none of these centers is near you, check your local newspapers and telephone directory. Or contact the American Society of Anesthesiologists (ASA), 515 Busse Highway, Park Ridge, Ill. 60068 (312) 825-5586. For a complete list of pain centers in the United States, request a copy of the ASA's pain clinic directory.

Pain Center
100 South Raymond
Alhambra, Calif. 91801

Pain Treatment Center
Hospital of Scripps Clinic
La Jolla, Calif. 92037

Pain Clinic
University of California Hospital
San Francisco, Calif. 94122

Pain Center
University of Miami
Miami, Fla. 33136

Emory University Pain Control Center
1441 Clifton Road, NE
Atlanta, Ga. 30322

Pain Clinic
University of Illinois College of Medicine
840 South Wood Street
Chicago, Ill. 60612

Pain Control Center
Mercy Hospital
New Orleans, La. 70119

Pain Treatment Center
Johns Hopkins University Medical School
Baltimore, Md. 21205

Boston Pain Unit
Massachusetts Rehabilitation Hospital
125 Nashua Street
Boston, Mass. 02144

Pain Clinic
Sister Kenny Institute
2727 Chicago Avenue
Minneapolis, Minn. 55404

Pain Management Center
Mayo Clinic–St. Mary's Hospital of Rochester
Rochester, Minn. 55901

Pain Treatment Center
Montefiore Hospital and Medical Center
Bronx, N.Y. 10467

Nebraska Pain Management Center
University of Nebraska College of Medicine
42nd Street and Dewey Avenue
Omaha, Neb. 68105

Ohio Pain and Stress Center
1460 West Lane Avenue
Columbus, Ohio 43221

Northwest Pain Center
10615 SE Cherry Blossom Drive
Portland, Ore. 97216

Pain Clinic
University of Virginia Medical Center
Charlottesville, Va. 22903

Pain Clinic
John J. Bonica, Director
University of Washington Medical School
Seattle, Wash. 98195

FOR MORE INFORMATION

For pain research:

• *PRN Forum* (a bimonthly newsletter)
Center for Health Sciences
Department of Anesthesiology
600 Highland Avenue
Madison, Wis. 53792

• *Office of Scientific Health Reports*
National Institute of Neurological and Communicative Disorders and Stroke
Building 31, Room 8A06
National Institutes of Health
9000 Rockville Pike
Bethesda, Md. 20205

• *National Health Information Clearinghouse* (sponsored by the Office of Disease Prevention and Health Promotion, U.S. Department of Health and Human Services)
For health information, call:
(800) 336-4797 (outside Virginia)
(703) 522-2590 (from Virginia)
For drug abuse information, call:
(800) 638-2045 (outside Maryland)
(800) 492-2948 (from Maryland)

The following organizations can also supply information:

• American Pain Society
70 West Hubbard Street
Chicago, Ill. 60610

• International Association for the Study of Pain
Department of Anesthesiology, RN-10
University of Washington
Seattle, Wash. 98195

• National Committee on the Treatment of Intractable Pain
P.O. Box 9553
Friendship Station
Washington, D.C. 20016-1553

APPENDIX

McGILL COMPREHENSIVE PAIN QUESTIONNAIRE ©

To be completed by the person with pain

1. PAIN HISTORY

- When did this pain begin?

Year: ________ Month: ________

- Did this pain begin:

gradually ________ suddenly ________

- How did this pain begin? Please check (√), then give more specific details on the lines below.

☐ Accident at work
☐ Accident at home
☐ Following an illness
☐ Following surgery
☐ Pain just began
☐ Other (e.g., car accident) ________

____

- Were there any changes in your life during the year before this pain began? (e.g., job change, buying or selling a home, death or loss of a friend or family member, marital problems) ________

____

____

- Is the pain the same now as it was when it began? Yes ☐ No ☐

2. PAIN TREATMENTS

Please place a check (√) in the box before any of the professionals you have consulted for the pain problem.

☐ Acupuncturist
☐ Allergist
☐ Anesthesiologist
☐ Cardiologist
☐ Chiropractor
☐ Clergyman
☐ Dentist
☐ Dermatologist
☐ Ear-nose-throat specialist
☐ Endocrinologist
☐ Faith healer
☐ General practitioner
☐ Gynecologist/obstetrician
☐ Hypnotist
☐ Internist
☐ Neurologist
☐ Neurosurgeon
☐ Nurse
☐ Oncologist
☐ Ophthalmologist
☐ Orthopedist
☐ Osteopath
☐ Pain clinic
☐ Pediatrician
☐ Physiatrist
☐ Physiotherapist
☐ Plastic surgeon
☐ Proctologist
☐ Psychiatrist
☐ Psychologist
☐ Radiologist
☐ Rheumatologist
☐ Social worker
☐ Surgeon (general)

Please list all the treatments you have had and are currently having for your pain. Include operations, hospitalizations, anesthetic procedures, physiotherapy and psychological treatments:

Name and type of specialist ________

____

____

Date started ________

Type of treatments and number of treatments (for example, once a week/every day) ________

____

Helped ________

____

Did not help ________

____

3. PAST MEDICAL HISTORY

Please list any illnesses *other than your pain problem* that you have had *at any age.* Also include allergies, hospitalizations, operations, anesthetic procedures, physiotherapy, and psychological illnesses and/or treatments. Please make an (×) beside any painful condition.

____

____

____

____

4. PRESENT MEDICAL HISTORY

- Please list any illnesses or health problems (other than the pain problem) you may have *now,* (e.g., high blood pressure, ulcer, etc.)

Problem ________

Present treatment ________

- Are you still menstruating?

Yes ☐ No ☐

If yes, is there any effect on the pain problem? Yes ☐ No ☐

5. MEDICATION

Please read the following list of drugs below and on page 121 carefully. Place a check (√) in the box beside any drug you have used for any reason. If you have taken a drug for pain: please mark in the box a + if it increased pain; please mark a − if it lessened the pain; please mark a 0 if it did not help; if you are allergic to any of these drugs please mark it with an A.

☐ acetaminophen
☐ Alka-Seltzer
☐ Anacin
☐ Ascriptin
☐ Aspirin
☐ Atasol**
☐ Atasol with codeine**
☐ Bufferin
☐ Darvon*
☐ Darvon mixtures*
☐ Entrophen**
☐ Equagesic
☐ Execedrin
☐ Fiorinal*
☐ Fiorinal with Codeine
☐ Frosst 217**
☐ Frosst 222*
☐ Frosst 282*
☐ Frosst 642*
☐ Frosst 692*
☐ Propoxyphene
☐ Tylenol
☐ Tylenol with codeine*
☐ Demerol
☐ Dilaudid
☐ heroin

*Not available in Canada
**Not available in the United States

Source: Monks, R., and Taenzer, P. "A Comprehensive Pain Questionnaire," in *Pain Measurement and Assessment,* edited by R. Melzack. New York: Raven Press, 1983. Reprinted with permission of the publisher.

- ☐ methadone
- ☐ morphine
- ☐ Paregoric
- ☐ Percodan*
- ☐ Talwin
- ☐ Butazolidin
- ☐ Clinoril*
- ☐ dexamethasone
- ☐ Feldene*
- ☐ hydrocortisone
- ☐ Indocid*
- ☐ Malgesic**
- ☐ Motrin
- ☐ Nalfon
- ☐ Naprosyn
- ☐ prednisolone
- ☐ prednisone
- ☐ Tandearil*
- ☐ Tolectin
- ☐ Arlidin
- ☐ Cafergot*
- ☐ Ergotrate
- ☐ Gynergen
- ☐ Inderal
- ☐ Sandomigran**
- ☐ Sansert
- ☐ Vasodilan
- ☐ Dantrium
- ☐ Flexeril
- ☐ meprobamate
- ☐ Norgesic*
- ☐ Robaxin
- ☐ Soma
- ☐ Ativan
- ☐ diazepam
- ☐ Equanil*
- ☐ Librium
- ☐ Miltown
- ☐ Serax
- ☐ Tranxene
- ☐ Valium
- ☐ Vivol**
- ☐ Amytal
- ☐ Butisol*
- ☐ Nembutal
- ☐ phenobarbital
- ☐ Seconal*
- ☐ Benadryl
- ☐ chloral hydrate
- ☐ Dalmane
- ☐ Doriden
- ☐ Halcion
- ☐ L-Tryptophan
- ☐ Noludar
- ☐ Paraldehyde
- ☐ Periactin
- ☐ Placidyl
- ☐ amitriptyline
- ☐ Anafranil**
- ☐ Aventyl
- ☐ doxepin
- ☐ Elavil
- ☐ Etrafon*
- ☐ lithium
- ☐ Ludiomil*
- ☐ Marplan
- ☐ Nardil
- ☐ Norpramin
- ☐ Parnate
- ☐ Pertofrane
- ☐ Sinequan
- ☐ Tofranil
- ☐ Triavil*
- ☐ Vivactil*
- ☐ Atarax
- ☐ Haldol
- ☐ Largactil**
- ☐ Mellaril
- ☐ Moditen**
- ☐ Navane
- ☐ Phenergan
- ☐ Sparine
- ☐ Stelazine
- ☐ Trilafon
- ☐ amphetamines
- ☐ hashish
- ☐ LSD
- ☐ marijuana
- ☐ mescaline
- ☐ phencylidine (PCP)
- ☐ Dexedrine
- ☐ Ionamin
- ☐ Ritalin
- ☐ Tenuate
- ☐ Tenuate Dospan
- ☐ Dilantin
- ☐ Tegretol penicillins
- ☐ erythromycin
- ☐ Keflex
- ☐ tetracycline
- ☐ multivitamins
- ☐ vitamin A
- ☐ vitamin B
- ☐ vitamin C
- ☐ vitamin D
- ☐ vitamin E
- ☐ vitamin K
- ☐ birth control pill
- ☐ other ______________

Please list *ALL* drugs you are *NOW* taking for any reason, including drugs which MAY NOT be on the list, whether prescribed by a doctor or not (include home remedies, over-the-counter medications, birth control pills).

Name of drug ______________

____

Dosage ______________

____

How many times per day/per week ______________

Reason for taking ______________

____

____

6. ACCOMPANYING SYMPTOMS

Please read the following list carefully. If you have *any* of these symptoms, *with your pain,* mark it with *W.P.* If you have them at *other times,* mark it with *O.T.*

- ______ Blurred vision
- ______ Constipation
- ______ Cough
- ______ Diarrhea
- ______ Difficulty breathing
- ______ Difficulty urinating
- ______ Dizziness
- ______ Excessive sweating
- ______ Numbness at nonpain sites
- ______ Fainting
- ______ Fatigue
- ______ Headache
- ______ Itching
- ______ Memory loss
- ______ Nasal stuffiness
- ______ Nausea
- ______ Rash
- ______ Ringing in the ear(s)
- ______ Swelling of tissues
- ______ Skin color change
- ______ Skin temperature change
- ______ Tearing of eyes
- ______ Vomiting
- ______ Weakness
- ______ Other ______________

CONTINUED ON PAGE 122

APPENDIX CONTINUED

McGILL COMPREHENSIVE PAIN QUESTIONNAIRE © CONTINUED

7. PAIN DESCRIPTION

Using the body figures shown below, please mark in *with a pencil* the areas where you feel the pain.

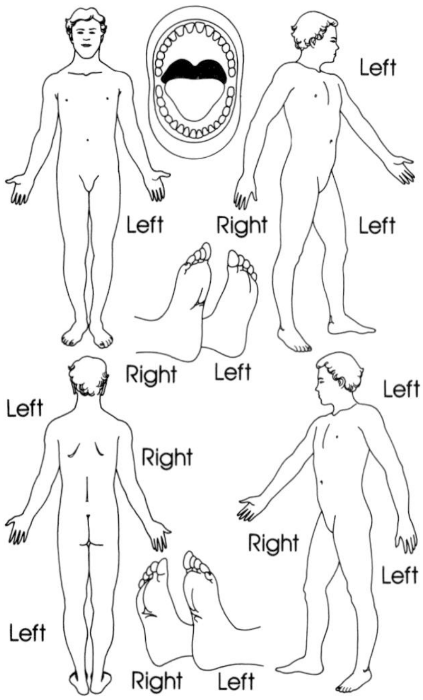

Left Right Left Left Right Left Left Right Left Right Right Left Left Right Left

8. TIME PATTERN DURING THE DAY

- Do you have the pain immediately on waking? Yes ☐ No ☐
If no, when does the pain begin?
______
______
______

- Does the pain change during the day? Yes ☐ No ☐
If yes, what part of the day is the pain *worse?* ______
What part of the day is the pain *better?* ______
- How many hours of the day are you *in pain?* ______
- How many hours of the day are you *pain-free?* ______

9. PAIN MODIFIERS

- For each of the following: Please mark with a + if it increases the pain; please mark with a − if it decreases the pain; please mark with a 0 if it has no effect on the pain.

☐ Bright lights
☐ Casts
☐ Cold
☐ Collars
☐ Corsets
☐ Coughing, sneezing
☐ Going to toilet
☐ Heat
☐ Housework
☐ Loud noises
☐ Lying
☐ Massage
☐ Mild exercise
☐ Sitting
☐ Standing
☐ Vibrator
☐ Vigorous exercise
☐ Walking
☐ Weather
☐ Work related
☐ Others ______
______
______
______

- Using the same signs (+, −, 0) as in the above question, please indicate how any of the following feelings and social situations affect your pain.

☐ Anger
☐ Being with others
☐ Contentment
☐ Enjoying things
☐ Fatigue
☐ Frustration
☐ Happiness
☐ Sadness
☐ Talking with others
☐ When others are sympathetic

- If parts of your body (e.g., stomach or muscles) are tense or tight, does the pain get worse?
Yes ☐ No ☐
Which parts of your body get tense or tight? ______
- Have you found that pain changes when you are with certain people (e.g., relatives, boss, etc.)? Yes ☐ No ☐ If yes, please specify: ______
- Does rest decrease your pain? Yes ☐ No ☐ How many hours do you rest each day? ______
Where and how do you usually rest? ______
- Have you learned any *specific* ways to relax yourself when the pain is bad? Yes ☐ No ☐ If yes, what do you do? ______
- How do people around you know that you are in pain? ______

10. EFFECTS OF PAIN

Work

- At what age did you start working full-time? ______
- How many jobs have you had?
______
- What is the longest length of time you have held a job? ______
- What type of work do you do or did you do last (include housework)? ______
______

For how long? ______
Number of hours per week ______
Duties (particularly physical activities, body postures, emotional stresses) ______
______

- Has the pain caused any change in your work?
Yes ☐ No ☐
If yes, do the changes include:
Change in number of hours worked? Yes ☐ No ☐
from ______hours per week before to ______hours per week now
Change of type of work?
Yes ☐ No ☐ from ______to ______
______

Satisfaction with work?
more ☐ same ☐ less ☐
Efficiency at work?
more ☐ same ☐ less ☐
Change in how you get/got along with co-workers, clients, etc?
Yes ☐ No ☐
If yes, please specify: ______
______

- Was/is your salary adequate for what you did/do? Yes ☐ No ☐
In general, before the pain began,

did your employer treat you fairly? Yes ☐ No ☐
Since the pain began?
Yes ☐ No ☐
If no, please specify: ______

• *If you are not working presently:* If you did not have a pain problem would you go back to work? Yes ☐ No ☐
• What job would you really like to have? ______

Finances
• Are you receiving any income for your disability? Yes ☐ No ☐
If yes, from whom (i.e. workman's compensation, pension, insurance) ______
When did this begin? ______
When will it be stopped? ______
Do you feel it is adequate?
Yes ☐ No ☐ Specify: ______
• Number of individuals on family income: ______
Who is the main contributor to this income? ______
Do others contribute?
Yes ☐ No ☐ Which others? ______
Since when? ______
• Do you have any debts?
Yes ☐ No ☐
Are you in financial need?
Yes ☐ No ☐
If yes, what steps have you taken to correct this? ______
• Do you have health insurance?
Yes ☐ No ☐ Details: ______

Legal proceedings *(litigation)*
• Are you involved in a lawsuit concerning the pain? (Specify: Lawyer, against whom, what are you requesting) ______
• Have you been involved in a legal suit in the past?
Yes ☐ No ☐ Results: ______

Leisure
• Are there any hobbies, sports, recreational and social activities that you no longer do because of the pain? Yes ☐ No ☐
If yes, what activities? ______
• What hobbies, social activities, etc. do you still do? ______
• Do any of your present activities help take your mind off the pain? Yes ☐ No ☐ If yes, which ones? ______
• Are there any new activities that you have begun since the pain began? Yes ☐ No ☐ If yes, what activities? ______

Sleep
• When do you usually go to bed at night? ______
• Approximately how long does it take to fall asleep? ______
• Do you have trouble falling asleep? Yes ☐ No ☐
• What body position do you use to sleep? ______
• Do you awaken in the night?
Yes ☐ No ☐ How many times? ______ What hours? ______
Do you empty your bladder?
Yes ☐ No ☐
Do you take medication?
Yes ☐ No ☐
Do you awaken others?
Yes ☐ No ☐
If yes, what do they do? ______
When do you finally awaken for the day? ______
• Do you feel refreshed or worse in the morning? ______
• Was your sleep pattern different before the pain? Yes ☐ No ☐
If yes, please specify ______

Weight/diet
How is your appetite? Too good ☐
Good ☐ Poor ☐ Very poor ☐
• Has your weight changed since the pain began? Yes ☐ No ☐
If yes, from ______ lb or ______ kilos to ______ lb or ______ kilos
Have you dieted? Yes ☐ No ☐
Are you now? Yes ☐ No ☐
What is your weight now? ______
Your height? ______

Habits
• Do you smoke? Yes ☐ No ☐
If yes, what/how much? ______
• Please indicate the number of cups/bottles you drink of the following each day:
coffee ______ tea ______
cola ______
• Do you drink alcohol?
Yes ☐ No ☐ If yes, what type of alcoholic beverage(s)? ______
How much do you drink per day? ______
Do you drink to: relieve the
pain? Yes ☐ No ☐,
relax? Yes ☐ No ☐,
sleep? Yes ☐ No ☐,
socialize? Yes ☐ No ☐
• Have you had any problems because of alcohol (e.g., physical, legal, psychological, social)?
Yes ☐ No ☐ If yes, please explain (e.g., loss or difficulty with friends, family, job, liver disease, blackouts, passing out, seizures, fits, hallucinations, etc.): ______

PERSONAL HISTORY

Parents
• Were you adopted?
Yes ☐ No ☐ Your age at the time ______
• Has either of your parents died? Yes ☐ No ☐
If yes, please indicate: which parent, his/her age at the time, your age at the time, and the cause of death ______

CONTINUED ON PAGE 124

APPENDIX CONTINUED

McGILL COMPREHENSIVE PAIN QUESTIONNAIRE © CONTINUED

• Please indicate with a check in the appropriate boxes if any of these words apply to your mother or father.

Mother	Father	
☐	☐	Sad
☐	☐	Happy
☐	☐	Loving
☐	☐	Unloving
☐	☐	Rejecting
☐	☐	Accepting
☐	☐	Rewarding
☐	☐	Punishing
☐	☐	Satisfying
☐	☐	Frustrating
☐	☐	Sickly
☐	☐	Healthy
☐	☐	Supportive
☐	☐	Critical
☐	☐	Selfish
☐	☐	Giving
☐	☐	Honest
☐	☐	Dishonest
☐	☐	Cooperative
☐	☐	Competitive
☐	☐	Encouraging independence
☐	☐	Overprotective
☐	☐	Intrusive
☐	☐	Allows privacy
☐	☐	Authoritarian
☐	☐	Democratic
☐	☐	Easygoing
☐	☐	Strict

Other words you feel apply to mother or father ______________

____

Siblings

• Do/did you have any brothers or sisters? Yes ☐ No ☐

• If yes, how many brothers and sisters do/did you have? ________

• Where do you fit in the birth order (i.e., first, last, etc.)? ______

• If any brothers or sisters have died please indicate: which ones, their age at the time, your age at the time, and the cause of death ______________

____

____

____

Personal details

• Check (√) any of the following that applied to you during your childhood.

☐ Bed wetting
☐ Cruel to animals
☐ Destructive
☐ Extremely shy
☐ Fears
☐ Finicky with food
☐ Nail biting
☐ Withdrawn
☐ Fire setting
☐ Happy
☐ Hostile
☐ Like to play with others
☐ Lying
☐ Night terrors
☐ No friends
☐ Overactive
☐ Stammering
☐ Teeth grinding
☐ Temper tantrums
☐ Thumb sucking
☐ Unhappy
☐ Others ______________

• Please check (√) any of the following describing your school experience.

☐ Afraid to attend
☐ Enjoyed school
☐ Frequent absenteeism
☐ Frequent discipline
☐ Suspended
☐ Picked on
☐ Alone
☐ Shy
☐ Joined group activities
☐ Athletic
☐ Leader

Grades:

☐ Superior
☐ Very good
☐ Fair
☐ Poor
☐ Very poor
☐ Others ______________

• Which of the following describe your friendship patterns? Please check (√)

☐ Anxiety with others
☐ Avoid groups
☐ Loner
☐ Difficulty keeping friends
☐ No good friends
☐ Sociable
☐ Join groups
☐ Leader
☐ Follower
☐ Have good friends
☐ Long friendships
☐ Can share thoughts/feelings with others
☐ Date(d) opposite sex
☐ Enjoy(ed) dating opposite sex
☐ Other ______________

____

Do you daydream? Yes ☐ No ☐
Dream at night? Yes ☐ No ☐

Marriage

• Please check (√) and, if relevant, indicate the length of time you have been:

☐ Married ______________
☐ Remarried ______________
☐ Common law ______________
☐ Separated ______________
☐ Single ______________
☐ Living together ______________
☐ Divorced ______________
☐ Widowed ______________

• What is your partner's occupation? ______________

Children

• Please give the following information regarding your children:

Sex ______________
Age ______________
Living at home or away ________
Achievement(s)/problems ______

• Have you had any miscarriages? Yes ☐ No ☐

Dates: ______________

Did you have any aftereffects (medical or psychological)? ______

____

Others in home

• Are there any others who are regular members of the household? Yes ☐ No ☐

Details: ______________

____

____

REFERENCES AND ACKNOWLEDGMENTS

Books

Angevine, Jay B., Jr., and Cotman, Carl W. *Principles of Neuroanatomy.* New York: Oxford University Press, 1981.

Bresler, David E., and Trubo, Richard. *Free Yourself from Pain.* New York: Simon & Schuster, 1979.

Chusid, Joseph G. *Correlative Neuroanatomy and Functional Neurology,* 18th ed. Los Altos, Calif.: Lange Medical Publications, 1982.

Crue, Benjamin, Jr., ed. *Chronic Pain: Further Observations from City of Hope National Medical Center.* New York: SP Medical & Scientific Books, 1979.

Fagerbaugh, Shizuko, and Strauss, Anselm. *Politics of Pain Management: Staff-Patient Interaction.* Menlo Park, Calif.: Addison-Wesley Publishing Co., 1977.

Foley, K., and Sundaresas, N. *Cancer: Principles and Practice of Oncology,* edited by Vincent T. Devita, Jr. and Samuel Hellman. Philadelphia: J.B. Lippincott Co., 1982.

Gilman, Alfred G., et al., eds. *Goodman and Gilman's The Pharmacological Basis of Therapeutics,* 6th ed. New York: Macmillan Publishing Co., 1980.

Hackett, Thomas P., and Cassem, Ned H. *Massachusetts General Hospital Handbook of General Hospital Psychiatry.* St. Louis: C.V. Mosby Co., 1978.

Harwood, A. *Ethnicity and Medical Care.* Cambridge, Mass.: Harvard University Press, 1981.

Jacox, Ada. *Pain: A Sourcebook for Nurses and Other Professionals.* Boston: Little, Brown & Co., 1977.

Krieger, Dolores. *The Therapeutic Touch: How to Use Your Hands to Help or to Heal.* Englewood Cliffs, N.J.: Prentice-Hall, 1979.

McCaffery, Margo. *Nursing Management of the Patient with Pain,* 2nd ed. Philadelphia: J.B. Lippincott Co., 1979.

Melzack, Ronald, and Wall, Patrick D. *The Challenge of Pain.* New York: Basic Books, 1983.

Mitchell, George, and Mayor, Donald. *Essentials of Neuroanatomy,* 4th ed. New York: Churchill Livingstone, 1983.

Petrie, Asenath. *Individuality in Pain and Suffering.* Chicago: University of Chicago Press, 1978.

Sternbach, Richard A., ed. *The Psychology of Pain.* New York: Raven Press Publications, 1978.

Periodicals and Pamphlets

Alberico, Jane G. "Breaking the Chronic Pain Cycle," *American Journal of Nursing* 84:1222-25, October 1984.

Barber, Joseph. "Hypnosis As a Psychological Technique in the Management of Cancer Pain," *Cancer Nursing* 1:361-63, October 1978.

Boguslawski, M. "Therapeutic Touch: A Facilitator of Pain Relief," *Topics in Clinical Nursing* 2:27-37, April 1980.

Bruegel, M.A. "Relationship of Preoperative Anxiety to Perception of Postoperative Pain," *Nursing Research* 20:26-31, January/February 1971.

Chapman, C. Richard, and Bonica, John J. "Acute Pain." *Current Concepts.* The Upjohn Company, 1983.

Davitz, L.J., and Sameshima, Y. "Suffering As Viewed in Six Different Cultures," *American Journal of Nursing* 76:1296-97, August 1976.

Fultz, J.M., et al. "When a Narcotic Addict Is Hospitalized," *American Journal of Nursing* 80:478-81, March 1980.

Graber, R.F. "How the Pain Clinics Manage Pain," *Patient Care* 18(2):81-98, January 30, 1984.

Jacox, A.K. "Assessing Pain," *American Journal of Nursing* 79:895-900, May 1979.

Johnson, M. "Pain: How You Know It's There and What Do You Do?" *Nursing76* 6:48-50, September 1976.

Leporati, N.C., and Chychula, L.H. "How You Can Really Help the Drug-Abusing Patient," *Nursing82* 12:46-49, June 1982.

Maguire, L.C., et al. "Prevention of Narcotic Induced Constipation," *New England Journal of Medicine* 305(27):1651, December 31, 1981.

McCaffery, M. "Understanding Your Patient's Pain," *Nursing80* 10:26-31, September 1980.

Shealy, C.N. "Holistic Management of Chronic Pain," *Topics in Clinical Nursing* 2:1-8, April 1980.

Storlie, F. "Pointers of Assessing Pain," *Nursing78* 8:37-39, May 1978.

Terzian, Maureen P. "Neurosurgical Interventions for the Management of Chronic Intractable Pain," *Topics in Clinical Nursing* 2:75-88, April 1980.

We'd like to thank the following people for their help with this book:

JOHN F. BARNES, RPT
Chief Physical Therapist
Pain and Stress Control Center
Paoli, Pa.

JO ELAND, RN, PhD
(Eland Color Tool)
Assistant Professor of Nursing
College of Nursing
University of Iowa
Iowa City

GEORGE HEIDRICH, RN, MA
Department of Anesthesiology
Center for Health Sciences
Madison, Wis.

JOSEPH R. WALKER
Product Director
Codman & Shurtleff, Inc.
Randolph, Mass.

We'd also like to thank the following companies:

ABBOTT LABORATORIES
Abbott Park, Ill.

CORMED, INC.
Medina, N.Y.

INFUSAID CORPORATION
Norwood, Mass.

INDEX

A

Acetaminophen, 80
Acupressure, 63
Acupuncture
  basics, 62
  noninvasive types, 63
  uses for, 63
Acute pain, 6
Addiction, narcotic, 87
Adjuvants
  specific drugs and uses for, 93-94
  types of, 92
  See also specific drugs.
Afferent nerve fibers, defined, 8
Agonists. *See* Narcotic analgesics. *See also specific drugs.*
Agonist-antagonists. *See* Narcotic analgesics. *See also specific drugs.*
Algogenic substances. *See* Pain regulators.
Amitriptyline, 94
Analgesia, 97
Analgesics
  administration routes, 98
  adverse effects, 82, 84-85
  basics, 76-77
  commonly used NSAIDs, 80-81

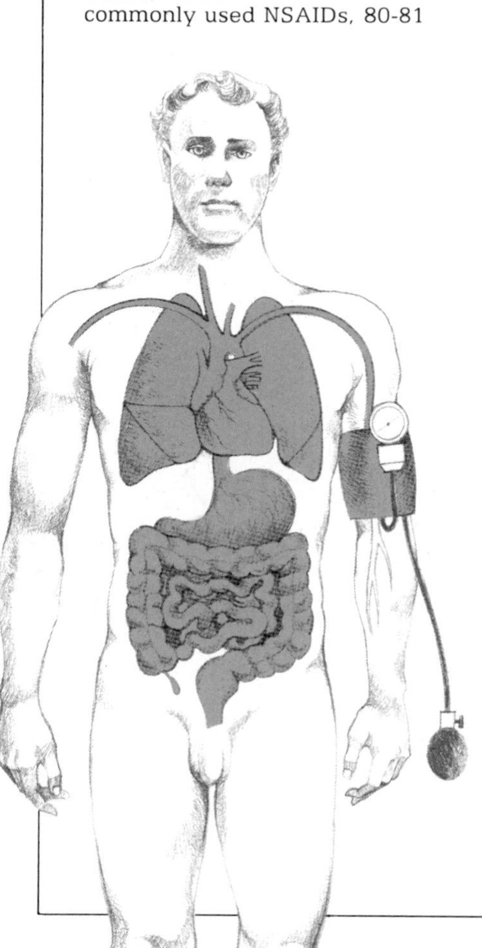

Analgesics *cont'd.*
  dosage schedules, 98
  guidelines for use, 78-80
  interactions, 82
  modifying analgesic therapy, 99
  myths about, 77
  naloxone, to reverse respiratory depression, 84
  narcotic analgesics, 83
  pediatric considerations, 116-117
  potencies of, 100
  respiratory depression, from narcotic analgesics, 83-84
Anticonvulsant drugs, 93
Antihistamines, 93
Antipsychotic drugs, 93
Aspirin, 80
Assessment, pain
  adults, 26-36
  children, 111-115
Axon, defined, 8

B

Back rub. *See* Massage.
Behavior modification. *See* Nonpharmacologic interventions.
Benzodiazepines, 94
Biofeedback, 60-61
Buprenorphine hydrochloride, 89
Butorphanol tartrate
  dosages and routes, 91
  facts about, 88

C

Carbamazepine, 93
Care plans for pain management, 36
Chiropractic. *See* Nonpharmacologic interventions.
Chlorpromazine, 93
Chronic pain
  definition of, 6
  patient's emotional response to, 24
Cingulotomy, 69
Clonazepam, 93
Codeine
  dosages and routes, 90
  facts about, 88
Cold laser therapy, 63
Cold therapy
  basics, 52-53
  combined with contralateral stimulation, 54
  guidelines, 53
  ice therapy, 53
Continuous infusion. *See* Infusion systems.
Cordotomy, 67-68

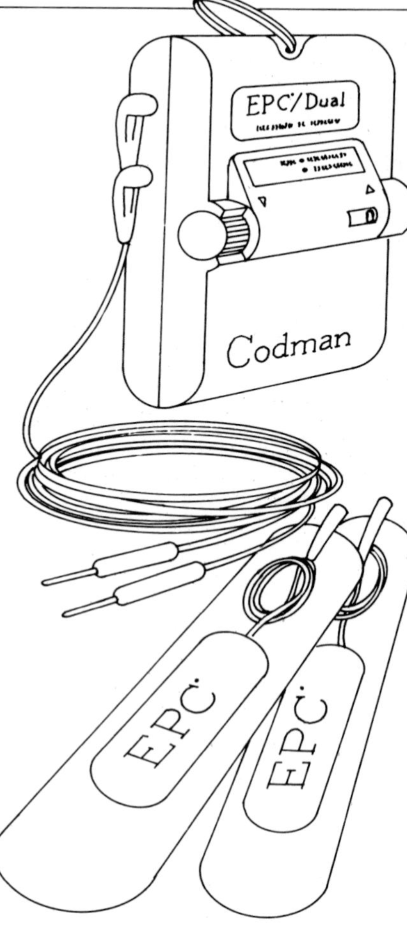

D

Dendrites, defined, 8
Dermatome, defined, 8
Distraction
  basics, 44
  guidelines for using, 46
  techniques, 45
Dorsal horn, defined, 8
Dorsal root entry zone (DREZ) lesion, 69
Doxepin, 94
Drugs, action of. *See* Pharmacokinetics.

E

Efferent nerve fibers, defined, 8
Eland color tool, 114-115
Electrical stimulation. *See* Transcutaneous electrical nerve stimulation.
Electronic acupuncture, 63
Endogenous opioids. *See* Endorphins.
Endorphins, 14-15

Epidural analgesia, 104-106
Equianalgesia, 99-100

Faith healing. *See* Nonpharmacologic interventions.
Fluphenazine, 93

Gate control theory of pain, 16-17
Goals for pain management, 32
Guided imagery
  basics, 48
  guidelines, 49

Haloperidol, 93-94
Heat therapy
  deep heat, 52
  guidelines, 52
  superficial heat, 51-52
Heroin, as therapeutic option, 89
Hydromorphone hydrochloride
  dosages and routes, 90
  facts about, 88
Hydroxyzine, 93
Hypnosis
  basics, 50
  myths about, 50
  techniques, 51
Hypophysectomy, 68

Ibuprofen, 80
Imipramine hydrochloride, 94
Implantable infusion systems. *See* Infusion systems.
Infusion systems, 102-106

Johnson's two-component scales. *See* Pain assessment tools.

Laser therapy. *See* Cold laser therapy.
Levorphanol tartrate
  dosages and routes, 90
  facts about, 88
Limbic system, defined, 8

Massage
  basics, 55
  myofascial release, 55
  techniques, 55-56
McGill Comprehensive Pain Questionnaire, 120-124
Menthol treatments, 54
Meperidine hydrochloride
  dosages and routes, 90
  facts about, 88
Methadone hydrochloride
  dosages and routes, 90
  facts about, 88
Methylphenidate hydrochloride, 94
Morphine
  dosages and routes, 91
  facts about, 87
  pediatric considerations, 117
Myofascial release. *See* Massage.

N

Nalbuphine hydrochloride
  dosages and routes, 91
  facts about, 88
Naloxone, to reverse narcotic-induced respiratory depression, 84
Narcotic analgesics
  administration guidelines, 89
  adverse effects, 83-85
  tolerance/dependence, 86
  types of, 88
  See also specific drugs.
Neospinothalamic tract. *See* Pain pathways.
Nerve blocks, 66-67
Neurectomy, 68
Neuroglial cells, 10
Neuron, anatomy of, 8-10
Neurosurgical procedures. *See* Surgical procedures for pain relief.
Neurotransmitters. *See* Pain regulators.
Nociceptors, 10
Nonpharmacologic interventions
  acupuncture, 62-63
  behavior modification, 64-65
  biofeedback, 60-61
  chiropractic, 64-65
  cold therapy, 52-54
  developing a pain-relief program, 38-40
  distraction, 44-46
  faith healing, 65
  guided imagery, 48-49
  heat therapy, 51-52
  hypnosis, 50-51
  massage, 55-56
  menthol treatments, 54
  nerve blocks, 66-67
  orgone therapy, 65
  patient teaching, 43-44
  pediatrics, 118
  relaxation, 46-47
  rolfing, 65
  surgical procedures, 67-69
  therapeutic touch, 65
  transcutaneous electrical nerve stimulation (TENS), 57-59
  tryptophan supplements, 65

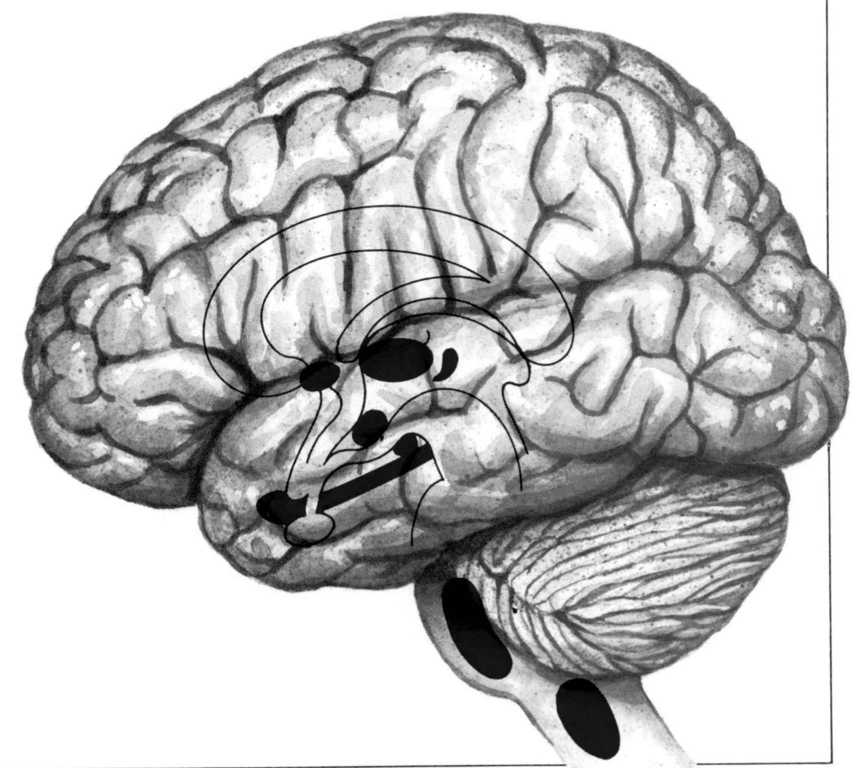

INDEX

Nonsteroidal anti-inflammatory drugs (NSAIDs)
  administration of, 83
  adverse effects, 81-82
  basics, 78-79
  interactions, 82
  specific drugs, 80-81
NSAIDs. *See* Nonsteroidal anti-inflammatory drugs.

Orgone therapy. *See* Nonpharmacologic interventions.
Over-the-counter drugs, 80
Oxycodone hydrochloride
  dosages and routes, 91
  facts about, 88
Oxymorphone, 100

Pain
  assessment of, 26-32
  basic concepts, 6-7
  cultural influences, 21
  familial influences, 21
  miscellaneous influences, 21-22
  myths about, 23
  patient's interpretation of, 20
  pediatric considerations, 108-118
  personal attitudes, 23
  personality influences, 19
  psychologic component of, 19
  sociocultural influences, 22
  stereotyping, 21
  theories, 16-17
  transmission of, 12-13
Pain assessment tools, 34-35
  for adults, 33-35, 120-124
  for children, 111-115
Pain-control centers, 70-72
Pain pathways, 12-13
Pain regulators, 12
Pain response, stages, 19
Pain sites, 7
Pain transmission
  pathways, 12-13
  prostaglandins, 12
  regulators, 12
Paleospinothalamic tract. *See* Pain pathways.
Patient-controlled analgesia. *See* Infusion systems.
Patient teaching, taking medication, 101
Pattern theory of pain, 16
Pediatrics
  analgesic administration, 116
  basics, 108
  morphine, dosages and routes, 117
  myths about, 108-110
  nonpharmacologic interventions, 118
  pain and developmental stage, 112-113
  pain-rating tools, 114
  pain response, 111-112
Pentazocine
  dosages and routes, 91
  facts about, 88
Pharmacokinetics
  drug absorption, 74
  drug distribution, 75
  drug excretion, 76
  drug metabolism, 75
Placebos, 94-97
Play therapy. *See* Therapeutic play.
Propoxyphene hydrochloride
  dosages and routes, 91
  facts about, 88
Prostaglandins, 12
Psychosocial influences in pain, 20-24

Referred pain, 18
Relaxation
  basics, 46-47
  progressive muscle relaxation, 47
  relaxation response, 47
Respiratory depression, as adverse effect of narcotic analgesia, 83-84
Rhizotomy, 68
Rolfing. *See* Nonpharmacologic interventions.

Specificity theory of pain, 16
Spinal cord, role in pain transmission, 10-11
Stewart pain circles. *See* Pain assessment tools.
Stewart pain color scale. *See* Pain assessment tools.
Stimulants, 94
Strong agonists. *See* Narcotic analgesics.
Surgical procedures for pain relief, 67-69.
Sympathectomy, 68

T

TENS. *See* Transcutaneous electrical nerve stimulation.
Therapeutic play, 118
Therapeutic touch. *See* Nonpharmacologic interventions.
Tractotomy, 69
Transcutaneous electrical nerve stimulation (TENS), 57-59
Tricyclic antidepressants, 94
Tryptophan supplements. *See* Nonpharmacologic interventions.

Weak agonists. *See* Narcotic analgesics. *See also specific drugs.*

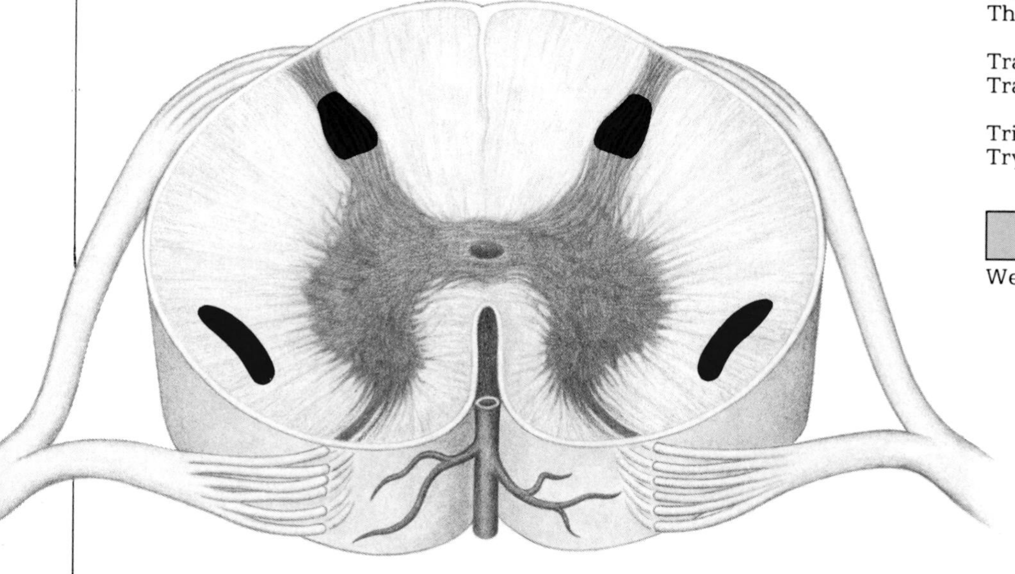